The Global Burden of Stroke and Changing Risk Factors

Edited by Serefnur Ozturk

Published in London, United Kingdom

The Global Burden of Stroke and Changing Risk Factors
http://dx.doi.org/10.5772/intechopen.1005947
Edited by Serefnur Ozturk

Contributors
Abdul Hanif Khan Yusof Khan, Anusha Thomas, Ashish Sharma, Ayotomiwa Fagbemi, Ayush Agarwal, Bao Minh Ton Luu, Bogdan Ciopleias, Changyang Zhong, Cong Wu, Guochu Peng, Huiming Dou, Jingxin Zhang, Maria Khan, Mirjam R. Heldner, Neetika Sharma, Olaleye Akinmola Adeniji, Rajeshwar Sahonta, Sarah Shali Matuja, Selam Kifelew, Tamer Roushdy, Thien Tan Tri Tai Truyen, Wei Zhu, Yinquan Sun, Yong Lu, Zhang Zuyong, Zhe Kang Law

First published in London, United Kingdom, 2025 by IntechOpen
IntechOpen is the global imprint of INTECHOPEN LIMITED, registered in England and Wales, registration number: 11086078, 167-169 Great Portland Street, London, W1W 5PF, United Kingdom

For EU product safety concerns: IN TECH d.o.o., Prolaz Marije Krucifikse Kozulić 3, 51000 Rijeka, Croatia, info@intechopen.com or visit our website at intechopen.com.

British Library Cataloguing-in-Publication Data
A catalogue record for this book is available from the British Library

The Global Burden of Stroke and Changing Risk Factors
Edited by Serefnur Ozturk
p. cm.
Print ISBN 978-1-83634-875-7
Online ISBN 978-1-83634-874-0
eBook (PDF) ISBN 978-1-83634-876-4

Meet the editor

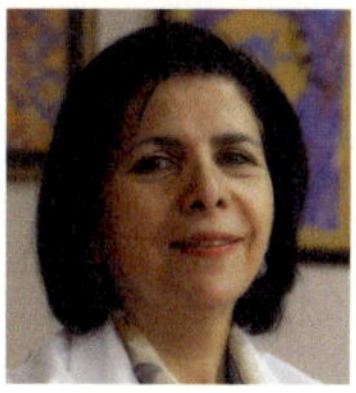

Serefnur Ozturk is Professor of Neurology and Head of the Neurology Department and Stroke Center of Selcuk University, Faculty of Medicine in Konya, Türkiye. She is past president of The Turkish Neurological Society and member of many national and international committees (WSO Global Policy Committee, Chair of WFN Migrant Neurology Specialty Group, EANcore CoVID-19 Task Force, European Academy of Neurology (EAN) Rare Diseases, Vice President of the WFN Environmental Specialty Group, UEMS Representative of Turkey and Secretary General of UEMS/EBN, member of UEMS /Neurology Section, Board Examination Committee, Co-president of the EAN Critical Care Panel, The Committee of Quality in Stroke Care –Turkish Health Ministry, executive board member of The Cerebrovascular Disease and Neurointensive Working Group of The Turkish Neurological Society. Her interests are stroke, neurointensive care, neuroepidemiology, health care, and neurological education. She has participated in the national and international phase III and IV projects and registries (as national coordinator and investigator). She is a member of TurkStrokeNet (Collaborate with ESOTA). She has more than 150 national and international publications (including books). Prof. Ozturk served as Editor-in-Chief of The Turkish Journal of Neurology and as a Board Member-Reviewer for more than 15 national and international journals.

Contents

Preface

Stroke remains one of the most complex and multifaceted health problems facing modern medicine. A leading cause of mortality and morbidity worldwide, this disease is a global public health problem that profoundly impacts individuals' quality of life, places a significant burden on healthcare systems, and has the potential to alter the socioeconomic balance of societies. Despite scientific advances, advanced imaging methods, and increasingly robust intervention strategies, the burden of stroke remains persistent in many regions and is increasingly prevalent, particularly in low- and middle-income countries. This book, titled "The Global Burden of Stroke and Changing Risk Factors", aims to meticulously analyze current data, trends, and predictions regarding stroke on a global scale. The subsequent section, which examines regional differences and region-specific risk factors, strikingly demonstrates how inequalities in access to healthcare and cultural and socioeconomic dynamics shape stroke burden. The chapters specifically addressing the impact of socioeconomic inequalities on stroke reveal a broader problem that must be addressed not only at the medical, but also at the societal and political levels. One of the most striking aspects of the book is its comprehensive coverage of the increasingly important topic of stroke in young people. The epidemiology, etiology, and risk management of stroke in young people demonstrate that contemporary lifestyle changes are leading to serious cerebrovascular consequences, even in young people. This content is a critical guide not only for clinicians but also for health policymakers, rehabilitation specialists, and public health researchers. The stroke risk presented in the final chapter highlights the preventable nature of the disease and reiterates the crucial role of early diagnosis, monitoring, and appropriate management strategies in reducing the burden of stroke. This approach is a key component of the evidence-based prevention, early intervention, and comprehensive management trilogy that permeates the book.

This book offers a holistic view of stroke, examining it not only as a clinical presentation but also as a multilayered phenomenon encompassing biological, environmental, economic, and social aspects. Each chapter, prepared by leading researchers in the field, brings together current, reliable, and in-depth information needed by both the academic world and clinical practice. I hope this book will provide new perspectives for all professionals, researchers, and health policymakers working in the fight against stroke, and contribute to the development of more effective prevention strategies, more equitable healthcare services, and stronger public awareness.

I sincerely congratulate all the authors, researchers, and scientists who contributed to this valuable work.

Serefnur Ozturk
Faculty of Medicine,
Department of Neurology,
Selcuk University,
Konya, Turkey

Chapter 1

Global Burden of Stroke: Insights and Trends from GBD 2021

Bao Minh Ton Luu and Thien Tan Tri Tai Truyen

Abstract

Stroke represents a major global health challenge, being one of the leading causes of death worldwide. In developed countries, while both the incidence and prevalence of stroke have generally declined, these nations now face the growing burden of stroke-related disability and the demands of post-stroke rehabilitation, exacerbated by an aging population and increasing life expectancy. In contrast, developing countries are confronting an even more challenging situation, as stroke rates are rising not only among the elderly but also among younger individuals, driven by the detrimental effects of modern lifestyles and environmental factors. Additionally, these nations struggle with significant challenges in managing and treating stroke, largely due to limited healthcare resources. This chapter aims to provide a comprehensive analysis of the global burden of stroke, highlighting the disparities in prevention, treatment, and care strategies, as well as the long-term impacts of the disease in both developed and developing nations.

Keywords: stroke, epidemiology, global burden disease, mortality, risk factor, LMICs

1. Introduction

Stroke, defined as "rapidly developing clinical signs of focal (or global) disturbance of cerebral function, lasting more than 24 hours or leading to death, with no apparent cause other than that of vascular origin" [1], remains one of the leading causes of death worldwide. According to data from the Global Burden of Disease (GBD). In 2021 there were 93.8 million (95% Uncertainty Interval [UI]: 89.0–99.3) stroke survivors, 11.9 million (10.7–13.2) new stroke events, 7.3 million (6.6–7.8) deaths attributed to stroke, and 160.5 million (147.8–171.6) Disability-Adjusted Life Years (DALYs) lost due to stroke. These figures accounted for 10.7% (9.8–11.3) of all deaths and 5.6% (5.0–6.1) of total DALYs from all causes, ranking stroke as the third leading cause of death, and the fourth leading cause of DALYs, after COVID-19 and ischemic heart disease. Notably, 83.3% of incident strokes, 76.7% of prevalent strokes, 87.2% of stroke-related deaths, and 89.4% of stroke-related DALYs occurred collectively in low- and middle-income countries (LMICs) [2]. A global meta-analysis conducted in 2011 estimated the pooled cumulative risks of stroke recurrence as 3.1% (95% CI: 1.7–4.4) at 30 days, 11.1% (95% CI: 9.0–13.3) at 1 year, 26.4% (95% CI:

20.1–32.8) at 5 years, and 39.2% (95% CI: 27.2–51.2) at 10 years following the initial stroke event [3]. Given the high mortality rates, substantial DALYs, and notable recurrence risk, stroke profoundly impacts individual health and results in enduring psychological, social, and economic consequences. These severe outcomes escalate pressures on social development and healthcare systems, particularly within countries that have limited resources.

In 2019, the global value of lost welfare (VLW) due to stroke was estimated at US$2059.67 billion, corresponding to 1.66% of global Gross domestic product (GDP) [4]. The economic impact is particularly severe in Central European, Eastern European, and Central Asian regions, where the VLW-to-GDP ratio reached 3.01% [4]. Beyond direct costs related to emergency services, acute care, and rehabilitation, indirect costs, including productivity loss, long-term disability, and informal caregiving, account for approximately 32% of the total economic burden of stroke and are projected to increase further with the population aging and improved post-stroke survival [5]. Notably, lifetime indirect costs per patient have been estimated to reach as high as US$54,067, with informal caregiving accounting for up to 80% of these costs. Stroke survivors often face persistent disabilities impairing mobility, communication, and self-care, leading to long-term dependence on caregivers [5]. A study of 22,929 patients revealed that 70–79% were either deceased or dependent at five years post-stroke [6]. Moreover, psychological sequelae are highly prevalent, with cognitive impairment affecting 30.0% of survivors, depression at 39.1%, and anxiety at 34.9%, further diminishing quality of life [7].

2. Current burden of stroke

2.1 Global burden

In 2021, stroke was the third leading cause of death globally. Among the primary subtypes, ischaemic stroke accounted for the largest share of new cases (65.3% [62.4–67.7]), followed by intracerebral hemorrhage (28.8% [28.3–28.8]) and subarachnoid hemorrhage (5.8% [5.7–6.0]) [8]. Ischemic strokes result from blood vessel blockage, commonly due to large artery disease, arteriolosclerosis, or cardioembolism while hemorrhagic strokes occur due to blood vessel rupture, leading to intracerebral bleeding. Deep hemorrhages are typically associated with hypertension, while lobar hemorrhages may be related to amyloid angiopathy or vascular malformations.

Although hemorrhagic strokes are less common, they generally have a poor prognosis and account for a greater proportion of stroke-related DALYs (79.5 million, or 49.6%) than ischaemic stroke (70.4 million, or 43.8%) [9]. The risk of death from hemorrhagic stroke is up to four times higher in the first week, 2.5 times higher after 1 week, and 1.5 times higher after 3 weeks compared to ischemic stroke [10]. Significant geographic variation was observed in age-standardized stroke metrics. For instance, the lowest incidence was reported in Luxembourg (57.7 per 100,000 [95% UI: 53.5–62.1]), while the highest was observed in the Solomon Islands (355.0 per 100,000 [95% UI: 332.7–378.1]). Stroke prevalence was highest in Ghana (2045.8 per 100,000) and lowest in Cyprus (521.5 per 100,000), whereas age-standardized death rates ranged from 14.2 per 100,000 in Singapore to 277.4 per 100,000 in North Macedonia. The highest stroke burden, as measured by age-standardized incidence, prevalence, mortality, and DALYs, occurred in East Asia, Central Asia, and sub-Saharan Africa, and was lowest in high-income regions such as North America, Australasia, and Latin America [9].

Between 1990 and 2021, there was a significant global reduction in age-standardized stroke metrics: incidence decreased by 21.8% (95% UI –23.7 to −19.8), prevalence by 8.5% (−9.7 to −7.3), mortality by 39.4% (−44.0 to −34.6), and DALYs by 38.7% (−43.4 to −34.0). However, during the same period, the absolute number of stroke cases and outcomes increased: new stroke events rose by 70.2% (65.9 to 74.6), stroke survivors by 86.1% (83.0 to 89.4), stroke-related deaths by 44.1% (32.3 to 56.0), and stroke-related DALYs by 32.2% (21.7 to 42.7). Notably, the pace of decline in age-standardized stroke incidence slowed in recent years: −1.8% (−2.8 to −0.6) during 2019–2021, compared to −3.1% (−4.2 to −2.0) across 2010–2021 [9].

Among individuals aged ≥70 years, there were substantial reductions in stroke incidence (−18.2% [−21.3 to −14.6]), mortality (−34.2% [−39.4 to −29.3]), and DALY rates (−35.6% [−40.2 to −30.8]) from 1990 to 2021, while prevalence remained relatively unchanged (−1.0% [−3.1 to 1.2]). In contrast, among individuals aged <70 years, the stroke incidence increased by 4.1% (0.9 to 7.6), and prevalence rose by 14.8% (13.1 to 16.8). Death and DALY rates in this younger group decreased by 17.4% (−25.0 to −8.9) and 19.0% (−26.0 to −11.6), respectively. These trends were consistent across ischaemic stroke subtypes. However, the prevalence of subarachnoid hemorrhage in people under 70 years increased slightly by 3.4% (1.3 to 5.5), while the incidence, prevalence, mortality, and DALYs associated with intracerebral hemorrhage and subarachnoid hemorrhage declined in both age groups [9].

The observed divergence between declining age-standardized stroke rates and rising absolute numbers of stroke events, deaths, and DALYs reflects the complex interplay between epidemiological transition and demographic change. On one hand, substantial progress in primary prevention, such as improved blood pressure control, reductions in tobacco use, healthier diets, and expanded access to acute stroke care, has contributed to notable decreases in stroke incidence and mortality at the individual level. However, these gains are offset by rapid global population growth, particularly in LMICs [11], and by marked population aging worldwide. As the ≥70-year-old age group, those at highest risk for stroke, expands in both absolute and relative terms, the total number of stroke events continues to increase despite lower individual risk. Moreover, advances in acute stroke management have improved survival, resulting in a growing number of stroke survivors who live with long term disability, thereby sustaining or increasing total DALYs. This trend does not signify failure in stroke prevention, but rather highlights a shifting public health challenge: an aging population that is living longer, but with greater post-stroke care needs. The implications are particularly profound for LMICs, which face the dual burden of rising non-communicable diseases and limited health system capacity to manage long-term sequelae [12].

2.2 Low-and middle-income countries

Stroke remains a leading cause of death and disability globally, but its epidemiological burden and the quality of stroke care differ substantially between the high-income countries (HICs) and LMICs. Over recent decades, LMICs have accounted for the majority of new stroke events, stroke-related deaths, and DALYs lost globally [13–16]. According to the GBD Study 2021, LMICs contributed to 83.3% of incident strokes, 76.7% of prevalent stroke cases, 87.2% of stroke-related deaths, and 89.4% of total stroke DALYs. Significant differences in stroke subtype distributions also exist; ischemic stroke accounted for 74.9% (95% UI 72.3–84.1) of incident strokes in HICs, compared with only 63.4% (53.6–73.7) in LMICs. Conversely, intracerebral hemorrhage comprised a higher proportion of strokes in LMICs (31.1% [30.2–31.3]) than in HICs (17.8% [17.3–17.9]), reaching its highest proportion in low-income countries (36.9% [36.5–37.1]). Subarachnoid hemorrhage was more common in HICs (7.3% [7.2–8.3]) than LMICs (5.5% [5.4–5.7]) [2].

Socioeconomic status and health-system capacity significantly influence stroke outcomes. Individuals with lower socioeconomic status typically experience reduced access to high-quality acute and rehabilitation stroke care compared to their counterparts with higher socioeconomic status, resulting in poorer clinical outcomes [17]. Access to comprehensive stroke care, including stroke units, acute treatments, and rehabilitation services, varies substantially between HICs and LMICs. For instance, stroke units are available in approximately 91% of HICs, compared to only 18% of low-income countries. Similarly, the availability of acute stroke therapies is substantially greater in HICs (approximately 60%) than in low-income settings (approximately 26%) [18]. Furthermore, rehabilitation care, including inpatient and community-based services, is considerably less accessible in LMICs.

These disparities are clearly evident within continents, particularly across five major regions: Africa, South Asia, Southeast Asia, Oceania, and South America. In Africa, stroke incidence and prevalence remain consistently high, with annual incidence rates reaching up to 316 per 100,000 and prevalence up to 1460 per 100,000 [19]. Stroke fatality rates are alarmingly elevated, often exceeding 80% at 3 years post-stroke. Strokes in African populations occur at younger ages, amplifying their socioeconomic impact. Moreover, this burden is growing, driven by escalating rates of non-communicable diseases and inadequate control of hypertension [20]. South Asia and Southeast Asia, including India, have among the highest global age-standardized incidence, mortality, and DALY rates associated with stroke. Major risk factors in these regions include hypertension, diabetes, and tobacco use, with considerable inter-country variability observed. In South America, the stroke burden remains high yet highly heterogeneous, characterized by marked disparities in incidence rates and outcomes across countries. In Oceania, while comprehensive data are scarce, available evidence indicates significant within-region disparities [21]. Even within individual continents, stroke incidence, mortality, and disease burden remain substantially higher in LMICs compared with their neighboring high-income countries. In Africa, for instance, Nigeria reports a stroke prevalence of approximately 1.14 per 1000 population, with 30-day case fatality rates reaching as high as 40% [22]. The disability and mortality from stroke in Nigeria impose significant socioeconomic impacts, reflected by a stroke-related DALYs burden nearly sevenfold higher than in high-income regions [23]. Similarly, in South Asia, stroke ranks as the fourth leading cause of death and fifth leading cause of disability in India, with incidence rates ranging from 105 to 172 per 100,000 people annually, and prevalence between 26 and 757 per 100,000 [24]. One-month stroke case fatality rates in India vary from 18 to 42%, with hospitalization costs reaching up to INR 50,000, imposing substantial financial burdens and chronic disability on affected families [25]. Within Southeast Asia, stroke remains a major public health concern. In Vietnam had a considerably higher age-standardized stroke mortality rate of 196·56 per 100,000 (95% UI: 164·21–226·77). Despite this high burden, from 1990 to 2021, Vietnam experienced gradual reductions in stroke incidence, mortality, and DALYs, with average annual percentage changes (AAPCs) of −0·34%, −0·49%, and − 0·61%, respectively [26].

2.3 HIC versus LMICs

Although stroke is a global public health crisis, its burden is unequally distributed with LMICs bearing a disproportionately high share of cases, deaths, and disability. Approximately 86% of all stroke deaths and 89% of stroke-related DALYs occur in LMICs [27]. Over the past four decades, LMICs have experienced more than a two-fold increase in stroke incidence, in stark contrast to a 42% decline observed in HICs during the same period [28]. Furthermore, patients in LMICs typically experience stroke at significantly younger ages (63 years) compared to their HIC counterparts (69 years), resulting in a greater loss of productive life years and amplifying socioeconomic consequences [18]. The health system challenges in LMICs are profound when prehospital emergency systems are often underdeveloped, leading to delayed hospital arrival, and stroke units remain scarce, with only 18% of LMICs reporting dedicated stroke rehabilitation services compared to over 90% in HICs [29]. Access to essential acute interventions such as intravenous thrombolysis and mechanical thrombectomy remains severely restricted in LMICs, with thrombolysis administered to approximately 3% of eligible patients in these settings, in stark contrast to usage rates as high as 30–40% in advanced stroke centers within high-income countries [30]. Post-acute care is equally inadequate. Most LMIC stroke survivors lack formal rehabilitation services. They are cared for by family members without professional support, leading to higher rates of long-term disability and dependency [31]. As a result, stroke survivors in LMICs frequently endure persistent severe disabilities, poor quality of life, and perpetuate cycles of poverty and social isolation.

3. Risk factors for stroke

The factors influencing stroke risk can be broadly categorized into three major groups: behavioral factors, including genetic predisposition, ethnicity, lifestyle, and health-related behaviors; metabolic factors, encompassing underlying medical conditions such as hypertension and diabetes, as well as the capacity and responsiveness of the healthcare system; and environmental or occupational factors, such as air pollution and climate change, in which nonmodifiable risk factors for stroke include age, sex, race–ethnicity, and genetic predisposition. Stroke is predominantly a disease of aging, and national health systems should leverage these factors to identify vulnerable populations for targeted screening programs. However, these nonmodifiable factors should not be the central focus of stroke prevention strategies. Instead, greater attention must be directed toward modifiable risk factors. Evidence indicates that approximately 90% of the global stroke burden is attributable to a small number of potentially modifiable risk factors, and a growing body of research demonstrates that addressing these factors can lead to a substantial reduction in stroke incidence [32]. The INTERSTROKE study, a large international case–control investigation, identified ten modifiable risk factors significantly associated with ischemic stroke including hypertension, current smoking, elevated waist-to-hip ratio, poor dietary patterns, physical inactivity, diabetes mellitus, binge alcohol consumption, psychosocial stress and depression, cardiac disease, and an elevated apolipoprotein B to A1 ratio. For intracerebral hemorrhage, key modifiable risk factors included hypertension, smoking, high waist-to-hip ratio, unhealthy diet, and heavy alcohol use [33].

Although the importance of modifiable risk factors is consistently emphasized across all major stroke prevention guidelines worldwide, the real-world control of these factors remains suboptimal, particularly in LMICs, where healthcare systems often lack adequate capacity. Globally, in 2019, only approximately 23% of women and 18% of men with hypertension had their blood pressure controlled (<140/90 mmHg), with the highest rates (>50%) observed in high-performing countries such as South Korea, Canada, and Iceland. In contrast, many LMICs reported control rates below 10% [34]. Contributing barriers include poor hypertension detection, inadequate or insufficient therapy, limited access to medications, physician inertia, and low adherence among patients. The COVID-19 pandemic further disrupted screening and management efforts, exacerbating existing gaps in care [35, 36]. To address this, proposals have included the creation of a Global Hypertension Care Taskforce and the implementation of an "80–80–80" strategy, aiming for 80% of adults screened, 80% of those diagnosed receiving treatment, and 80% of treated patients achieving blood pressure control [37].

Similarly, while the global pooled rate of diabetes control improved from 16% before 2000 to 22% after 2010, significant disparities remain. Control rates are higher in high-income countries, whereas they remain as low as 16% in low-income settings [38]. Poor control of diabetes in LMICs can largely be attributed to the demanding nature of effective glycemic management, which requires strict medication adherence along with sustained dietary and physical activity modifications, practices that are difficult to maintain in contexts where health literacy is low and care-seeking behavior is predominantly symptom-driven. Furthermore, individuals in LMICs often face considerable financial and logistical barriers to accessing newer antidiabetic and antihypertensive agents, which have demonstrated superior efficacy and lower side-effect profiles compared to older treatments. Addressing these challenges will require a multifaceted response, including strengthening public health education and expanding government and global health support programs that improve access to affordable, effective therapies in resource-limited settings.

Another key determinant that contributes not only to stroke risk but also to the broader landscape of metabolic risk factors is the category of intrinsic factors, encompassing individual-level characteristics such as dietary habits, tobacco use, physical inactivity, and alcohol consumption. In 2010, the global mean sodium intake was estimated at 3.95 grams per day, with regional averages ranging from 2.18 to 5.51 grams. Sodium consumption above the recommended threshold was associated with approximately 1.65 million cardiovascular deaths annually (95% uncertainty interval: 1.10–2.22 million), accounting for 9.5% of all cardiovascular mortality worldwide. Among these, 61.9% occurred in men and 38.1% in women; notably, 84.3% of these deaths occurred in LMICs, and 40.4% occurred before the age of 70 [39]. Tobacco use remains a substantial public health concern, particularly in LMICs, which now account for the majority of the world's smokers. Smoking prevalence varies markedly across regions, from 13.5% in Africa to 32.2% in Asia [40], and a significant proportion in LMICs, between 7.5 and 38.4% of current smokers, are classified as "hardened smokers," defined as long-term daily users with low motivation to quit [41]. However, a range of tobacco control strategies have demonstrated real-world effectiveness in reducing tobacco use. Among these, fiscal measures, particularly taxation and price increases, are consistently identified as the most impactful interventions globally, with robust evidence supporting their role in curbing tobacco consumption and improving population-level health outcomes [42]. In parallel, legislative measures such as comprehensive bans on smoking in public places and workplaces have been shown to significantly reduce both smoking prevalence and exposure to secondhand smoke, and are widely endorsed as effective tools for governmental action [43].

Importantly, multi-component tobacco control programs that integrate taxation, regulatory policies, mass media campaigns, and cessation support are associated with greater reductions in tobacco use than single-strategy interventions, underscoring the value of comprehensive policy frameworks [44]. In addition, urbanization in LMICs is also contributing to a rise in sedentary behavior, particularly in densely populated urban centers [45]. Meanwhile, global obesity rates are accelerating more rapidly in LMICs than in high-income countries, especially among women and children [46]. While high-income countries have seen reductions in alcohol consumption driven by regulatory and public health measures, LMICs are experiencing a rise in alcohol use [47]. Heavy alcohol consumption contributes to elevated blood pressure, cardiac arrhythmias, and cardiomyopathy, all of which heighten the risk of stroke. Moreover, alcohol alters platelet function and coagulation pathways, thereby increasing the likelihood of both ischaemic and haemorrhagic events [48].

Environmental air pollution, particularly fine particulate matter ($PM_{2.5}$) and nitrogen dioxide (NO_2), is a well-established risk factor for both ischaemic and haemorrhagic stroke. Air pollution may precipitate cerebrovascular events through mechanisms involving inflammation, oxidative stress, and vascular dysfunction [49]. Both short-term and long-term exposures have been shown to increase stroke risk. Exposure to both fine ($PM_{2.5}$) and coarse (PM_{10}) particulate matter has been consistently associated with higher rates of stroke incidence, hospital admissions, and mortality. The association is particularly strong for $PM_{2.5}$ (OR = 1.008; 95% CI: 1.005–1.011) [50]. It is estimated that approximately 16.9% of the nearly 15 million strokes that occur annually worldwide can be attributed to air pollution, with both short- and long-term exposure contributing to increased risk, especially for strokes caused by atherosclerosis [51]. This burden is particularly pronounced in LMICs, where $PM_{2.5}$ concentrations are significantly higher. The annual mean exposure to $PM_{2.5}$ between 2011 and 2017 was 48.42 $\mu g/m^3$ in LMICs, compared to 20.02 $\mu g/m^3$ in HIC. $PM_{2.5}$ levels in many LMICs have been found to exceed WHO air quality standards and affect regions that collectively account for approximately 40% of the global population [52]. Effective air pollution control policies include comprehensive national plans such as China's Air Pollution Prevention and Control Action Plan, which set phased targets and cross-sector measures [53]; sector-specific interventions focusing on transportation, energy, and industry such as promoting public transit, transitioning to cleaner fuels, tightening emission standards [54], a combination of incentive-based and punitive approaches, including free public transportation, subsidies for clean household energy, and congestion pricing for vehicles [55]. These policies have contributed to significant reductions in $PM_{2.5}$, PM_{10}, and SO_2 levels, along with public health gains.

A growing environmental determinant of stroke risk, particularly in LMICs, is exposure to extreme ambient temperatures, which contribute to approximately 13% of cardiovascular deaths and 5.2% of global stroke mortality [56, 57]. A multinational analysis involving data on 3,443,969 ischemic and 2.454.267 hemorrhagic stroke deaths across 522 cities in 25 countries demonstrated a U-shaped association, indicating elevated stroke mortality at both temperature extremes [58]. Specifically, extreme cold significantly increased hemorrhagic stroke risk (RR = 1.49, 95%CI 1.40–1.58) compared to ischemic stroke (RR = 1.34, 95% CI 1.27–1.41), whereas extreme heat was predominantly associated with ischemic stroke (RR = 1.13, 95%CI 1.06–1.20) rather than hemorrhagic stroke (RR = 1.02, 95% CI 1.00–1.05). Socioeconomic context further modified these relationships: countries with lower GDP per capita experienced higher risks of heat-related hemorrhagic stroke mortality (RR = 1.08, 95%CI 1.02–1.15), whereas ischemic stroke risk due to heat was comparable across income levels. Mechanistically, cold exposure promotes vasoconstriction, hypertension, cholesterol crystallization, plaque instability, and hypothermia-associated bleeding, thereby increasing stroke risks [59, 60]. Conversely, heat exposure induces dehydration, hemoconcentration, sympathetic activation, and systemic inflammation via heat shock proteins, all exacerbating thrombotic and ischemic events [61, 62].

The distribution and control of stroke risk factors differ markedly between HICs and LMICs, driving much of the global disparity in stroke incidence and outcomes. Hypertension, the most significant modifiable risk factor for stroke globally, is particularly poorly controlled in LMICs, where it affects up to 64% of stroke patients and is a principal driver of the higher proportion of hemorrhagic strokes (about 20% in LMICs versus 10% in HICs) [31]. LMICs are experiencing a rapid increase in other vascular risk factors, including diabetes and obesity, driven by urbanization, dietary transitions toward high-salt and high-fat foods, and reduced physical activity [31]. Environmental exposures such as ambient and indoor air pollution further exacerbate stroke risk in these regions. Moreover, region-specific factors, including chronic infections such at HIV-associated vasculopathy in sub-Saharan Africa and genetic disorders like sickle cell disease, disproportionately affect younger individuals in LMICs, contributing to earlier stroke onset and greater loss of productive life years. The underdiagnosis and suboptimal treatment of atrial fibrillation and hypercholesterolemia in LMICs, partly due to limited healthcare infrastructure and lower awareness, also contribute to uncontrolled stroke risk [31].

4. Management and rehabilitation

Effective stroke management encompasses rapid prehospital recognition and response, timely hospital-based reperfusion therapies, organized stroke unit care, and comprehensive post-acute rehabilitation. While these components are routinely integrated into HICs, their implementation remains severely limited in LMICs, contributing to higher mortality and disability rates. In LMICs, public awareness of stroke symptoms is generally low, and emergency medical services (EMS) are often fragmented or underdeveloped, resulting in delayed hospital arrival. This delay is a major barrier to the use of reperfusion therapies. Intravenous thrombolysis, a cornerstone intervention shown to improve functional independence by up to 30%, is administered to only ~3% of eligible patients in LMICs, compared to up to 30–40% in HICs. Access to mechanical thrombectomy, which offers an additional 14–25% improvement in favorable outcomes for large vessel occlusions, is nearly absent in LMICs [28, 63]. In many countries LMICs, the treatment rate is below 1% due to a lack of essential infrastructure such as angiographic suites and trained neurointerventionalists [30].

Once patients reach hospital care, the availability of stroke units, a critical intervention shown to reduce mortality by 14% and improve functional outcomes, is extremely limited, reported in only 18% of LMIC hospitals versus over 90% in HICs [64]. The computed tomography scan (CTs) capabilities, essential for differentiating ischemic and hemorrhagic stroke, are often limited to urban tertiary centers in LMICs. Rural and peripheral hospitals frequently lack both CTs and MRI, leading to reliance on clinical assessment alone and increasing the risk of mismanagement. In-hospital care in LMICs often lacks essential supportive measures such as early mobilization, dysphagia screening, and prevention of complications, resulting in higher rates of preventable in-hospital morbidity and mortality [28].

Addressing these deficiencies requires targeted investment in health system infrastructure, including the development of EMS networks, expansion of stroke unit capacity, and provision of affordable neuroimaging. Capacity-building efforts should prioritize training multidisciplinary teams, including stroke neurologists, nurses, physiotherapists, and speech therapists. Innovative, cost-adapted approaches such as telemedicine networks, mobile stroke units, and regional stroke referral pathways are promising strategies to overcome geographical and resource barriers. Moreover, policy-level commitment is needed to subsidize critical therapies such as thrombolysis and thrombectomy and integrate stroke into national non-communicable disease strategies. Improving acute stroke management in LMICs is essential to reducing early mortality, minimizing disability, and alleviating the long-term socioeconomic burden of stroke.

In recent years, stroke diagnosis has undergone significant advancements driven by rapid progress in imaging technologies, molecular biology, and the integration of artificial intelligence, all aiming to optimize classification, management, and prognostication in stroke patients. One of the most notable developments is the widespread implementation of CT angiography (CTA) and CT perfusion (CTP) imaging, which enables the early identification of large-vessel occlusion and delineation of salvageable brain tissue. Landmark trials such as DAWN and DEFUSE-3 have demonstrated that patient selection based on perfusion imaging allows safe extension of the mechanical thrombectomy window up to 6–24 hours after symptom onset, with markedly superior functional outcomes at 90 days compared to medical therapy alone (49% with 13%) [65]. Similarly, the EXTEND trial showed that intravenous thrombolysis remains effective up to 9 hours from onset in patients selected by CTP [66]. These findings have been incorporated into international clinical guidelines since 2019–2021, establishing CTA and CTP as standard tools for assessing late-presenting stroke. Advanced MRI techniques such as diffusion-weighted imaging (DWI) and FLAIR have also contributed to extending treatment eligibility; notably, the WAKE-UP trial demonstrated that DWI–FLAIR mismatch can reliably identify patients with wake-up stroke suitable for thrombolysis [67]. In parallel, blood-based biomarkers, especially glial fibrillary acidic protein (GFAP), are emerging as promising tools for rapid differentiation between ischemic and hemorrhagic stroke. A prospective study involving 353 acute stroke patients revealed that GFAP levels <30 pg./mL had a negative predictive value of 100% for excluding intracerebral hemorrhage, while levels >200 pg./mL strongly suggested hemorrhagic stroke, with a positive predictive value of 90–95% [68]. These findings have direct clinical implications: a negative GFAP test may support the safe initiation of early thrombolytic therapy, whereas a positive result necessitates urgent blood pressure control or reversal of anticoagulation. In addition, AI is increasingly being applied as an effective supportive tool in the early diagnosis of stroke, helping to shorten alert times, accelerate inter-hospital transfers, and significantly reduce 'door-in-door-out' time. A study utilizing Canon Medical's AI platform on 100 stroke CT cases demonstrated that the AI system could process CTA images in just 60 seconds, much faster than the average interpretation time by radiologists, which is 395 seconds, with a sensitivity of 77% for detecting large vessel occlusions, compared to 87% for radiologists [69]. However, algorithmic transparency and medicolegal issues related to diagnostic errors remain unresolved challenges. Taken together, these innovations pave the way for faster and more targeted therapeutic decision-making.

Advances in diagnostic imaging have led to numerous therapeutic breakthroughs. Mechanical thrombectomy, once restricted to 6 hours post-onset, is now effective up to 24 hours in selected patients, thanks to advanced imaging that identifies viable penumbral tissue, as demonstrated in the DAWN and DEFUSE-3 trials. DAWN reported a 49% rate of functional independence at 90 days versus 13% with standard medical therapy [66]. Intravenous thrombolysis has also seen expanded indications, with the EXTEND trial showing efficacy up to 9 hours post-onset in patients selected by CT perfusion imaging [70]. In hemorrhagic stroke, blood pressure management has been refined, guided by imaging predictors such as the CTA "spot sign," which indicates risk of hematoma expansion. Surgical approaches have also advanced: early minimally invasive hematoma evacuation is under active evaluation in ICH, while aneurysm coiling and clipping in subarachnoid hemorrhage benefit from earlier and more precise CTA-based diagnosis [70]. Additionally, neuroprotective strategies, though historically unsuccessful, are experiencing renewed interest through trials targeting specific molecular pathways or patient subsets. These advances are undoubtedly beneficial for patients, but they may also contribute to the stark disparities in outcomes between HICs and LMICs. While patients in HICs benefit directly from these novel approaches, those in LMICs often face significant barriers to access and implementation due to technological limitations and financial constraints.

5. Policy suggestion for low- and middle-income countries

LMICs should prioritize the development of integrated and comprehensive stroke care systems. Public education campaigns are essential to enhance community recognition of early stroke symptoms, commonly summarized by the acronym FAST as facial drooping, arm weakness, speech difficulties, and the necessity of timely activation of emergency medical services. Such initiatives must emphasize the critical importance of seeking immediate medical attention to optimize the chances of receiving acute interventions within the therapeutic window. Concurrently, raising public awareness about the availability, efficacy, and safety of acute-phase interventions, particularly intravenous thrombolysis (tPA), may facilitate timely hospital presentation and improve patient eligibility for reperfusion therapies.

Robust emergency medical service systems, dedicated stroke units within regional hospitals, and affordable, accessible neuroimaging infrastructure are foundational components required for timely diagnosis and effective management. Additionally, implementing telemedicine programs and remote consultation networks can empower local healthcare providers to manage complex stroke cases efficiently, minimize delays associated with inter-hospital transfers, and enhance access to specialized neurological expertise in resource-constrained settings.

Governments play a pivotal role in facilitating these advancements through supportive health policy development, financial subsidies for essential diagnostic tools and treatments, and integration of stroke prevention strategies within national non-communicable disease frameworks. Efforts targeting modifiable risk factors must be embedded within primary healthcare systems and reinforced by evidence-based public health interventions promoting healthy lifestyle behaviors and addressing environmental determinants.

Establishing multidisciplinary stroke care teams, including neurologists, rehabilitation physicians, specialized nurses, physiotherapists, speech-language pathologists, and occupational therapists, in conjunction with telemedicine expansions and mobile stroke units is critical for addressing existing gaps in stroke management. Through the implementation of these comprehensive strategies, LMICs can substantially reduce stroke morbidity and mortality, enhance functional patient outcomes, and alleviate the significant socioeconomic burdens posed by stroke.

Access to modern stroke therapies, particularly intravenous thrombolysis (tPA), remains a significant challenge in low- and middle-income countries (LMICs), mainly due to financial barriers and stringent post-treatment monitoring requirements [71, 72]. The standard protocol for blood pressure monitoring in the first 24 hours after intravenous rtPA bolus is highly intensive, involving up to 36 measurements, posing considerable strain on healthcare resources, which are typically limited in LMIC settings. Various LMICs have implemented financial-support policies and have reported substantial initial successes. In Thailand, the rate of tPA usage increased notably from 0.38% in 2007 to 6.5% in 2012 following its inclusion in the universal healthcare coverage program [73]. In Brazil, policies offering free tPA raised its use from 1.3% in 2009 to 12.5% in 2019 and reduced 30-day mortality rates [74]. In China, expansion of the "Green Channel" hospital network and enhanced insurance reimbursement led to thrombolysis rates exceeding 15% in tertiary hospitals [75]. Recently, the OTIMIST main study proposed a simplified blood pressure monitoring protocol for mild-to-moderate stroke patients (NIHSS <10), reducing measurement frequency from 36 to 18 times without adversely impacting treatment outcomes, thus alleviating healthcare system strain while maintaining patient safety [76].

The Mobile Stroke Unit (MSU) is an innovative pre-hospital care model that functions as a mobile stroke hospital. It is equipped with a 32-slice CT scanner, cerebral vascular imaging systems, and telemedicine technology that enables remote consultation with neurologists [77]. This approach facilitates early diagnosis and intervention during patient transport. Several LMICs have reported successful implementation of the MSU model. In Thailand, a study of 978 acute ischemic stroke patients showed that those treated by MSU had the shortest door-to-needle time (20 minutes), the highest reperfusion therapy rate (56.8%), and significantly better outcomes (adjusted OR 2.15, 95% CI: 1.39–3.32) [78]. By significantly shortening onset-to-treatment time, MSUs have shown improved clinical outcomes compared to conventional ambulance transport.

6. Conclusions

In conclusion, stroke poses a major public health challenge worldwide and particularly in LMICs, significantly contributing to global morbidity and mortality. Addressing this issue effectively requires integrated stroke care systems, improved community awareness, robust emergency services, and expanded diagnostic capabilities. Strategic investment in healthcare infrastructure, telemedicine programs, and multidisciplinary stroke care teams can bridge current service gaps. Through supportive government policies and targeted preventive measures, LMICs can substantially reduce stroke burden, enhance patient outcomes, and decrease associated socioeconomic consequences.

Conflict of interest

The authors declare no conflict of interest.

Notes/thanks/other declarations

None.

Acronyms and abbreviations

LMICs	low- and middle-income countries
HICs	high income countries
GBD	global burden of disease
DALYs	total disability-adjusted life years
VLW	the global value of lost welfare
GDP	gross domestic product
WHO	World Health Organization
EMS	emergency medical services
CTA	CT angiography
CTP	CT perfusion
GFAP	glial fibrillary acidic protein

Author details

Bao Minh Ton Luu[1] and Thien Tan Tri Tai Truyen[2]*

1 Can Tho University of Medicine and Pharmacy, Can Tho, Vietnam

2 Faculty of Medicine, Nam Can Tho University, Can Tho, Vietnam

*Address all correspondence to: taitruyenmd@gmail.com

References

[1] Aho K, Harmsen P, Hatano S, Marquardsen J, Smirnov VE, Strasser T. Cerebrovascular disease in the community: Results of a WHO collaborative study. Bulletin of the World Health Organization. 1980;**58**(1):113-130

[2] Feigin VL, Stark BA, Johnson CO, Roth GA, Bisignano C, Abady GG, et al. Global, regional, and national burden of stroke and its risk factors, 1990-2019: A systematic analysis for the Global Burden of Disease Study 2019. The Lancet Neurology. 2021;**20**(10):795-820. DOI: 10.1016/S1474-4422(21)00252-0

[3] Mohan KM, Wolfe CD, Rudd AG, Heuschmann PU, Kolominsky-Rabas PL, Grieve AP. Risk and cumulative risk of stroke recurrence: A systematic review and meta-analysis. Stroke. 2011;**42**(5):1489-1494. DOI: 10.1161/strokeaha.110.602615

[4] Gerstl JVE, Blitz SE, Qu QR, Yearley AG, Lassarén P, Lindberg R, et al. Global, regional, and National Economic Consequences of stroke. Stroke. 2023;**54**(9):2380-2389. DOI: 10.1161/STROKEAHA.123.043131

[5] Joo H, George MG, Fang J, Wang G. A literature review of indirect costs associated with stroke. Journal of Stroke and Cerebrovascular Diseases. 2014;**23**(7):1753-1763. DOI: 10.1016/j.jstrokecerebrovasdis.2014.02.017

[6] Sennfält S, Norrving B, Petersson J, Ullberg T. Long-term survival and function after stroke. Stroke. 2019;**50**(1):53-61. DOI: 10.1161/STROKEAHA.118.022913

[7] Crichton SL, Bray BD, McKevitt C, Rudd AG, Wolfe CD. Patient outcomes up to 15 years after stroke: Survival, disability, quality of life, cognition and mental health. Journal of Neurology, Neurosurgery & Psychiatry. 2016;**87**(10):1091-1098

[8] Feigin VL, Brainin M, Norrving B, Martins SO, Pandian J, Lindsay P, et al. World Stroke Organization: Global stroke fact sheet 2025. International Journal of Stroke. 2025;**20**(2):132-144. DOI: 10.1177/17474930241308142

[9] Feigin VL, Abate MD, Abate YH, Abd ElHafeez S, Abd-Allah F, Abdelalim A, et al. Global, regional, and national burden of stroke and its risk factors, 1990-2021: A systematic analysis for the global burden of disease study 2021. The Lancet Neurology. 2024;**23**(10):973-1003. DOI: 10.1016/S1474-4422(24)00369-7

[10] Andersen KK, Olsen TS, Dehlendorff C, Kammersgaard LP. Hemorrhagic and ischemic strokes compared. Stroke. 2009;**40**(6):2068-2072. DOI: 10.1161/STROKEAHA.108.540112

[11] Ezeh AC, Bongaarts J, Mberu B. Global population trends and policy options. The Lancet. 2012;**380**(9837):142-148. DOI: 10.1016/S0140-6736(12)60696-5

[12] Tan MP. Healthcare for older people in lower and middle income countries. Age Ageing. 1 Apr 2022;**51**(4):afac016. DOI: 10.1093/ageing/afac016

[13] Feigin V, Forouzanfar M, Krishnamurthi R, Mensah G, Connor M, Bennett D, et al. Global and regional burden of stroke during 1990-2010: Findings from the global burden of disease study 2010. The Lancet. 2014;**383**:245-255. DOI: 10.1016/S0140-6736(13)61953-4

[14] Howard G, Thrift A, Pandian J, Liu L, Norrving B, Howard V, et al. Global stroke statistics 2022. International Journal of Stroke. 2022;**17**:946-956. DOI: 10.1177/17474930221123175

[15] Mensah G, Feigin V, Ng M, Parmar P, Chugh S, Naghavi M, et al. Global burden of stroke and risk factors in 188 countries, during 1990-2013: A systematic analysis for the global burden of disease study 2013. The Lancet Neurology. 2016;**15**:913-924. DOI: 10.1016/S1474-4422(16)30073-4

[16] Krishnamurthi RV, Feigin VL, Forouzanfar MH, Mensah GA, Connor M, Bennett DA, et al. Global and regional burden of first-ever ischaemic and haemorrhagic stroke during 1990-2010: findings from the Global Burden of Disease Study 2010. The Lancet Global Health. Nov 2013;**1**(5):e259-81. DOI: 10.1016/S2214-109X(13)70089-5. Epub 2013 Oct 24

[17] Marshall IJ, Wang Y, Crichton S, McKevitt C, Rudd AG, Wolfe CDA. The effects of socioeconomic status on stroke risk and outcomes. The Lancet Neurology. 2015;**14**(12):1206-1218. DOI: 10.1016/S1474-4422(15)00200-8

[18] Rahbar MH, Medrano M, Diaz-Garelli F, Gonzalez Villaman C, Saroukhani S, Kim S, et al. Younger age of stroke in low-middle income countries is related to healthcare access and quality. Annals of Clinical and Translational Neurology. 2022;**9**(3):415-427. DOI: 10.1002/acn3.51507

[19] Venketasubramanian N, Yoon B, Pandian J, Navarro J. Stroke epidemiology in South, East, and South-East Asia: A review. Journal of Stroke. 2017;**19**:286-294. DOI: 10.5853/jos.2017.00234

[20] Owolabi MO, Akarolo-Anthony S, Akinyemi R, Arnett D, Gebregziabher M, Jenkins C, et al. The burden of stroke in Africa: A glance at the present and a glimpse into the future. Cardiovascular Journal of Africa. 2015;**26**(2 Suppl 1):S27-S38. DOI: 10.5830/CVJA-2015-038

[21] Markus H. The global burden of stroke. International Journal of Stroke. 2023;**18**:632-633. DOI: 10.1177/17474930231181677

[22] Wahab K. The burden of stroke in Nigeria. International Journal of Stroke. 2008;**3**:290-292. DOI: 10.1111/j.1747-4949.2008.00217.x

[23] Adigwe G. Quality of life of stroke survivors in Nigeria (low-income country). Can outcome be predicted? The Journal of Clinical Hypertension. 2021;**23**:1459-1462. DOI: 10.1111/jch.14258

[24] Jones S, Baqai K, Clegg A, Georgiou R, Harris C, Holland E-J, et al. Stroke in India: A systematic review of the incidence, prevalence, and case fatality. International Journal of Stroke. 2021;**17**:132-140. DOI: 10.1177/17474930211027834

[25] Kalita J, Bharadwaz MP, Aditi A. Prevalence, contributing factors, and economic implications of strokes among older adults: A study of North-East India. Scientific Reports. 2023;**13**(1):16880. DOI: 10.1038/s41598-023-43977-z

[26] Truyen TTTT, Vo NLY, Vo QP, Phan TC, Le PNB, Nguyen H-DT, et al. Burden and risk factors of stroke in Vietnam from 1990 to 2021–A systematic analysis from global burden disease 2021. Journal of Stroke and Cerebrovascular Diseases. 2025;**34**(3):108241

[27] Feigin VL, Brainin M, Norrving B, Martins S, Sacco RL, Hacke W, et al. World Stroke Organization (WSO): Global stroke

fact sheet 2022. International Journal of Stroke. 2022;**17**(1):18-29. DOI: 10.1177/17474930211065917

[28] Taiwo O, Koko MK, Hakim E. Stroke units in low and middle income countries (LMICs) save lives: Application of the western model of stroke care. South Sudan Medical Journal. 2024;**17**(1):4-5

[29] Feigin VL, Owolabi MO, Feigin VL, Abd-Allah F, Akinyemi RO, Bhattacharjee NV, et al. Pragmatic solutions to reduce the global burden of stroke: A World Stroke Organization–2013; Lancet Neurology Commission. The Lancet Neurology. 2023;**22**(12):1160-1206. DOI: 10.1016/S1474-4422(23)00277-6

[30] Asif KS, Otite FO, Desai SM, Herial N, Inoa V, Al-Mufti F, et al. Mechanical thrombectomy global access for stroke (MT-GLASS): A mission thrombectomy (MT-2020 Plus) study. Circulation. 2023;**147**(16):1208-1220. DOI: 10.1161/CIRCULATIONAHA.122.063366

[31] Aderinto N, Olatunji G, Kokori E, Abraham IC, Ogieuhi IJ, Ogunbowale I, et al. Disparities in post-stroke rehabilitation: An African perspective. Discover Public Health. 2025;**22**(1):218. DOI: 10.1186/s12982-025-00622-6

[32] Markus HS, Brainin M, Fisher M. Tracking the global burden of stoke and dementia: World Stroke Day 2020. International Journal of Stroke. 2020;**15**(8):817-818. DOI: 10.1177/1747493020959186

[33] Boehme AK, Esenwa C, Elkind MSV. Stroke risk factors, genetics, and prevention. Circulation Research. 2017;**120**(3):472-495. DOI: 10.1161/CIRCRESAHA.116.308398

[34] Zhou B, Carrillo-Larco R, Danaei G, Riley L, Paciorek C, Stevens G, et al. Worldwide trends in hypertension prevalence and progress in treatment and control from 1990 to 2019: A pooled analysis of 1201 population-representative studies with 104 million participants. Lancet (London, England). 2021;**398**:957-980. DOI: 10.1016/S0140-6736(21)01330-1

[35] Stergiou G, Cho M, Williams B, Schutte A, Wainford R, Mooi C, et al. Addressing global disparities in blood pressure control: Perspectives of the International Society of Hypertension. Cardiovascular Research. 2022;**119**:381-409. DOI: 10.1093/cvr/cvac130

[36] Beaney T, Wang W, Schlaich M, Schutte A, Stergiou G, Alcocer L, et al. Global blood pressure screening during the COVID-19 pandemic: Results from the may measurement month 2021 campaign. Journal of Hypertension. 2023;**41**:1446-1455. DOI: 10.1097/HJH.0000000000003488

[37] Pickersgill S, Msemburi W, Cobb L, Ide N, Moran A, Su Y, et al. Modeling global 80-80-80 blood pressure targets and cardiovascular outcomes. Nature Medicine. 2022;**28**:1693-1699. DOI: 10.1038/s41591-022-01890-4

[38] Shahrestanaki E, Mohammadian Khonsari N, Seif E, Baygi F, Ejtahed HS, Sheidaei A, et al. The worldwide trend in diabetes awareness, treatment, and control from 1985 to 2022: A systematic review and meta-analysis of 233 population-representative studies. Frontiers in Public Health. 17 May 2024;**12**:1305304. DOI: 10.3389/fpubh.2024.1305304

[39] Mozaffarian D, Fahimi S, Singh GM, Micha R, Khatibzadeh S, Engell RE, et al. Global sodium consumption and death from cardiovascular causes. New England Journal of Medicine. 14 Aug 2014;**371**(7):624-634. DOI: 10.1056/NEJMoa1304127

[40] Stubbs B, Vancampfort D, Firth J, Solmi M, Siddiqi N, Smith L, et al. Association between depression and smoking: A global perspective from 48 low- and middle-income countries. Journal of Psychiatric Research. 2018;**103**:142-149. DOI: 10.1016/j.jpsychires.2018.05.018

[41] Yin S, Ahluwalia IB, Palipudi K, Mbulo L, Arrazola RA. Are there hardened smokers in low- and middle-income countries? Findings from the Global Adult Tobacco Survey. Tobacco Induced Diseases. 18 Feb 2019;**17**:11. DOI: 10.18332/tid/100631

[42] Jha P, Chaloupka F, Corrao M, Jacob B. Reducing the burden of smoking world-wide: Effectiveness of interventions and their coverage. Drug and Alcohol Review. 2006;**25**(6):597-609. DOI: 10.1080/09595230600944511

[43] Levy D, Chaloupka F, Gitchell J. The effects of tobacco control policies on smoking rates: A tobacco control scorecard. Journal of Public Health Management and Practice : JPHMP. 2004;**10**(4):338-353. DOI: 10.1097/00124784-200407000-00011

[44] Wakefield M, Chaloupka F. Effectiveness of comprehensive tobacco control programmes in reducing teenage smoking in the USA. Tobacco Control. 2000;**9**:177-186. DOI: 10.1136/tc.9.2.177

[45] Khaltaev N, Axelrod S. Countrywide "best buy" interventions for noncommunicable diseases prevention and control in countries with different level of socioeconomic development. Chronic Diseases and Translational Medicine. 2022;**9**:44-53. DOI: 10.1002/cdt3.49

[46] Ford N, Patel S, Narayan K. Obesity in low- and middle-income countries: Burden, drivers, and emerging challenges. Annual Review of Public Health. 2017;**38**:145-164. DOI: 10.1146/annurev-publhealth-031816-044604

[47] Walls H, Cook S, Matzopoulos R, London L. Advancing alcohol research in low-income and middle-income countries: A global alcohol environment framework. BMJ Global Health. 2020;**5**:e001958

[48] Hillbom M. Alcohol consumption and stroke: Benefits and risks. Alcoholism, Clinical and Experimental Research. 1998;**22**(Suppl. 7):352-358. DOI: 10.1097/00000374-199807001-00012

[49] Kulick ER, Kaufman JD, Sack C. Ambient air pollution and stroke: An updated review. Stroke. 2023;**54**(3):882-893. DOI: 10.1161/strokeaha.122.035498

[50] Niu Z, Liu F, Yu H, Wu S, Xiang H. Association between exposure to ambient air pollution and hospital admission, incidence, and mortality of stroke: An updated systematic review and meta-analysis of more than 23 million participants. Environmental Health and Preventive Medicine. 26 Jan 2021;**26**(1):15. DOI: 10.1186/s12199-021-00937-1

[51] Leira EC, Latorre JG. Ambient pollution and stroke. Neurology. 2022;**98**(24):1003-1004. DOI: 10.1212/WNL.0000000000200801

[52] Sharma S, Chandra M, Kota SH. Health effects associated with PM2.5: A systematic review. Current Pollution Reports. 2020;**6**(4):345-367. DOI: 10.1007/s40726-020-00155-3

[53] Liu W, Lei Y, Feng Y, Ning M, Sun Y, Wang J. Defending blue sky in China: Effectiveness of the "air pollution prevention and control action plan" on air quality improvements from 2013 to 2017. Journal of Environmental Management. 2019;**252**:109603. DOI: 10.1016/j.jenvman.2019.109603

[54] Wang S, Xing J, Zhao B, Jang C, Hao J. Effectiveness of national air pollution control policies on the air quality in metropolitan areas of China. Journal of Environmental Sciences. 2014;**26**(1):13-22. DOI: 10.1016/S1001-0742(13)60381-2

[55] Jafari AJ, Charkhloo E, Pasalari H. Urban air pollution control policies and strategies: A systematic review. Journal of Environmental Health Science and Engineering. 2021;**19**:1911-1940. DOI: 10.1007/s40201-021-00744-4

[56] Alahmad B, Khraishah H, Royé D, Vicedo-Cabrera AM, Guo Y, Papatheodorou SI, et al. Associations between extreme temperatures and cardiovascular cause-specific mortality: Results from 27 countries. Circulation. 2023;**147**(1):35-46

[57] Burkart KG, Brauer M, Aravkin AY, Godwin WW, Hay SI, He J, et al. Estimating the cause-specific relative risks of non-optimal temperature on daily mortality: A two-part modelling approach applied to the global burden of disease study. The Lancet. 2021;**398**(10301):685-697

[58] Alahmad B, Khraishah H, Kamineni M, Royé D, Papatheodorou SI, Vicedo-Cabrera AM, et al. Extreme temperatures and stroke mortality: Evidence from a multi-country analysis. Stroke. 2024;**55**(7):1847-1856. DOI: 10.1161/STROKEAHA.123.045751

[59] Hata T, Ogihara T, Maruyama A, Mikami H, Nakamaru M, Naka T, et al. The seasonal variation of blood pressure in patients with essential hypertension. Clinical and Experimental Hypertension Part A: Theory and Practice. 1982;**4**(3):341-354

[60] Kuneš J, Tremblay J, Bellavance F, Hamet P. Influence of environmental temperature on the blood pressure of hypertensive patients in Montreal. American Journal of Hypertension. 1991;**4**(5_Pt_1):422-426

[61] Stewart S, Keates AK, Redfern A, McMurray JJ. Seasonal variations in cardiovascular disease. Nature Reviews Cardiology. 2017;**14**(11):654-664

[62] Gaudio FG, Grissom CK. Cooling methods in heat stroke. The Journal of Emergency Medicine. 2016;**50**(4):607-616

[63] Khatib R, Arevalo YA, Berendsen MA, Prabhakaran S, Huffman MD. Presentation, evaluation, management, and outcomes of acute stroke in low- and middle-income countries: A systematic review and meta-analysis. Neuroepidemiology. 2018;**51**(1-2):104-112. DOI: 10.1159/000491442

[64] Kayola G, Mataa MM, Asukile M, Chishimba L, Chomba M, Mortel D, et al. Stroke rehabilitation in low- and middle-income countries: Challenges and opportunities. American Journal of Physical Medicine & Rehabilitation. 2023;**102**(2S Suppl. 1):S24-S32. DOI: 10.1097/phm.0000000000002128

[65] Nogueira RG, Jadhav AP, Haussen DC, Bonafe A, Budzik RF, Bhuva P, et al. Thrombectomy 6 to 24 hours after stroke with a mismatch between deficit and infarct. New England Journal of Medicine. 2018;**378**(1):11-21

[66] Ma H et al. Thrombolysis guided by perfusion imaging up to 9 hours after onset of stroke. The New England Journal of Medicine. 2019;**380**(19):1795-1803. DOI: 10.1056/NEJMoa1813046

[67] Zhang J, Ta N, Fu M, Tian FH, Wang J, Zhang T, et al. Use of DWI-FLAIR mismatch to estimate the onset time in wake-up strokes. Neuropsychiatric

Disease and Treatment. 2022;**18**:355-361. DOI: 10.2147/ndt.S351943

[68] Kumar A, Misra S, Yadav AK, Sagar R, Verma B, Grover A, et al. Role of glial fibrillary acidic protein as a biomarker in differentiating intracerebral haemorrhage from ischaemic stroke and stroke mimics: A meta-analysis. Biomarkers. 2020;**25**(1):1-8. DOI: 10.1080/1354750x.2019.1691657

[69] Temmen SE, Becks MJ, Schalekamp S, van Leeuwen KG, Meijer FJ. Duration and accuracy of automated stroke CT workflow with AI-supported intracranial large vessel occlusion detection. Scientific Reports. 2023;**13**(1):12551

[70] Streib C. Tenecteplase for acute ischemic stroke thrombolysis: Practical considerations and real-world implementation. Neurology. Clinical Practice. 2024;**14**(1):e200221. DOI: 10.1212/cpj.0000000000200221

[71] Ghandehari K. Barriers of thrombolysis therapy in developing countries. Stroke Research and Treatment. 2011;**2011**(1):686797

[72] de Souza AC, Sebastian IA, Zaidi WAW, Nasreldein A, Bazadona D, Amaya P, et al. Regional and national differences in stroke thrombolysis use and disparities in pricing, treatment availability, and coverage. International Journal of Stroke. 2022;**17**(9):990-996. DOI: 10.1177/17474930221082446

[73] Suwanwela NC. Stroke epidemiology in Thailand. Journal of Stroke. 2014;**16**(1):1-7. DOI: 10.5853/jos.2014.16.1.1

[74] Moro CH, Gonçalves AR, Longo AL, Fonseca PG, Harger R, Gomes DB, et al. Trends of the incidence of ischemic stroke thrombolysis over seven years and one-year outcome: A population-based study in Joinville, Brazil. Cerebrovascular Diseases Extra. 2013;**3**(1):156-166

[75] Wang Q, Wang Y, Wang Y, Bi Q, Zhang Q, Wang F. Impact of improved stroke green channel process on the delay of intravenous thrombolysis in patients with acute cerebral infarction during the COVID-19 pandemic: An observational study. Frontiers in Neurology. 2022;**13**:998134. DOI: 10.3389/fneur.2022.998134

[76] Anderson CS, Summers D, Ouyang M, Sui Y, Johnson B, Billot L, et al. Safety and efficacy of low-intensity versus standard monitoring following intravenous thrombolytic treatment in patients with acute ischaemic stroke (OPTIMISTmain): An international, pragmatic, stepped-wedge, cluster-randomised, controlled non-inferiority trial. The Lancet. 2025;**405**(10493):1909-1922. DOI: 10.1016/S0140-6736(25)00549-5

[77] Fassbender K, Walter S, Liu Y, Muehlhauser F, Ragoschke A, Kuehl S, et al. "Mobile stroke unit" for hyperacute stroke treatment. Stroke. 2003;**34**(6):e44-e4e

[78] Nilanont Y, Chanyagorn P, Shukij K, Pengtong W, Kongmuangpuk M, Wongmayurachat K, et al. Comparing performance measures and clinical outcomes between mobile stroke units and usual care in underserved areas. Neurological Sciences. 2023;**44**(4):1261-1271

Chapter 2

Regional Burden and Region-Specific Stroke Risk Factors in Lower and Middle-Income Countries

Zhe Kang Law, Sarah Shali Matuja, Mirjam R. Heldner, Tamer Roushdy, Ayush Agarwal, Maria Khan, Bogdan Ciopleias, Abdul Hanif Khan Yusof Khan and Selam Kifelew

Abstract

In this chapter, we outline the trends in incidence, prevalence, and the burden of stroke in developing countries (lower- and middle-income countries—LMICs) over recent decades. We highlight the changes in risk factors and types of stroke (ischemic vs. hemorrhagic) in LMICs, comparing them to high-income countries (HIC). We will also use statistics from specific countries as case examples. The lack of resources and its impact on stroke management will be discussed. The authors include stroke physicians who are part of the World Stroke Organization Future Leaders Program and have carried out quality improvement projects in Sub-Saharan Africa, among other initiatives.

Keywords: stroke, intracerebral hemorrhage, lower and middle-income countries, epidemiology, incidence, prevalence, DALYs, burden, risk factors, developing countries

1. Introduction

Stroke is among the top 10 most common causes of death globally, being the third after ischemic heart disease and COVID-19, and accounting for approximately 10% of deaths worldwide [1]. Stroke is the leading cause of death in upper-middle-income countries (UMIC), the second leading cause of death in low-income countries (LIC), and the third leading cause of death in lower-middle-income countries (LMIC) [1]. Low- and middle-income countries constitute 89% of the global stroke burden as of 2025 [2]. Therefore, understanding the epidemiology of stroke in low- and middle-income countries is crucial in planning for developing strategies to reduce the global stroke burden. In this chapter, we explore the epidemiology of stroke in

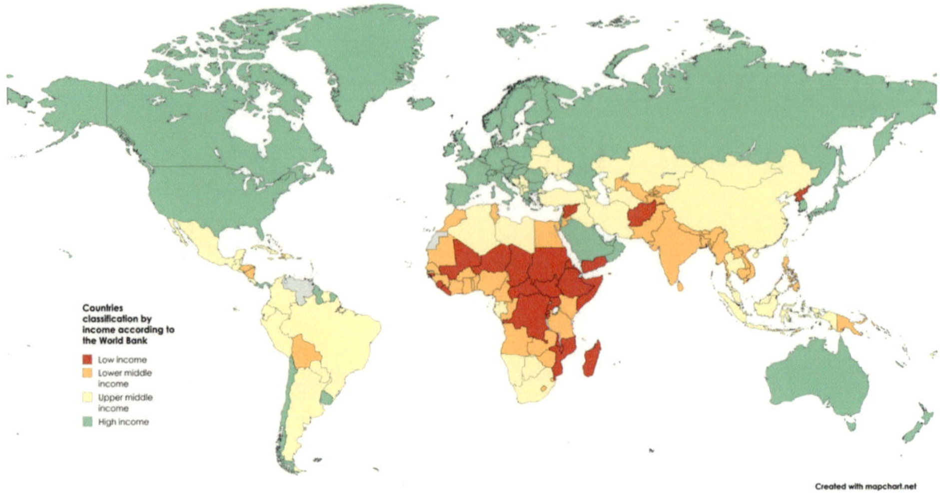

Figure 1.
Countries are classified by income according to the World Bank.

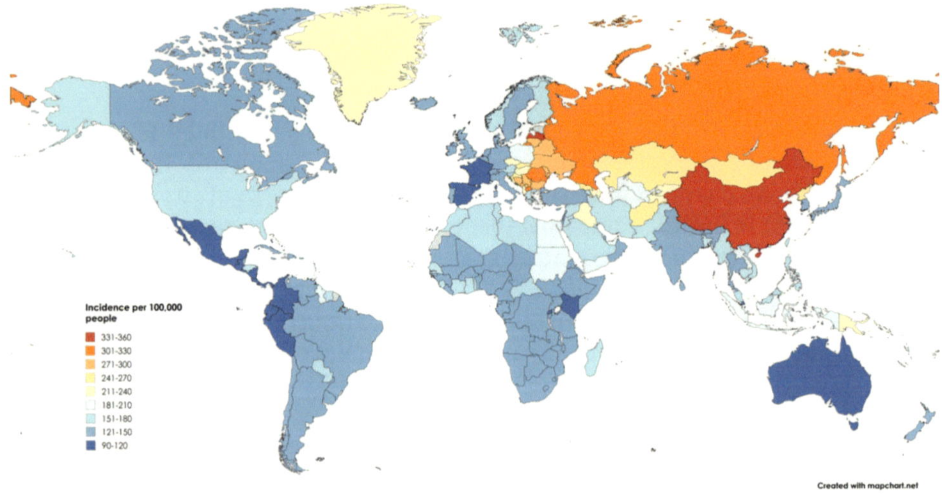

Figure 2.
Incidence of stroke per 100,000 population. Source: Adapted from Ref. [3].

a non-exhaustive list of low- and middle-income countries. A general overview of country classifications by income is provided in **Figure 1**, while **Figure 2** depicts the incidence of stroke worldwide.

2. Africa

2.1 Background

Africa is the second-largest and second most populous continent, consisting of 54 countries, an area of around 30 million km^2, and a population of around 1.2

billion. It is estimated to reach 2.2 billion for sub-Saharan Africa (SSA) by the year 2054 [4]. Africa's population is the youngest among the continents, with a median age of 19.7. Four African countries are densely populated with more than 100 million: Nigeria (>232 million), Ethiopia (>132 million), Egypt (>116 million), and the Democratic Republic of the Congo (>109 million), while the least populous country is Seychelles, with a population of around 130,000 [4].

Geographically, historically, religiously, and ecosystem, Africa is divided into two different regions, namely North Africa (NA), composed of five countries, and SSA, comprising the rest of the African countries [5]. NA countries are mostly inhabited by Arabic/Semitic as well as Berber ethnicity, while SSA has a diversity of ethnicities, with the majority classified as Niger-Congo and Nilo-Saharan [6, 7]. The World Bank classifies most African countries as low-income countries (LIC) and middle-income countries, except for Seychelles. These include seven upper-middle-income countries (UMIC), 22 lower-middle-income countries (LMIC), and 24 low-income countries (LIC) [5].

2.2 Burden of stroke

Africa's Daily Adjusted Life Years (DALYs) following stroke is around 17.3 million [2]. Although much lower than Asia's, the actual numbers might be higher, especially since the epidemiology of Africa is changing owing to socio-demographic changes with many countries shifting to urbanization and lifestyle changes with changes in modifiable and non-modifiable vascular risk factors [8, 9].

There is still a scarcity of epidemiological data in many African countries owing to deficiencies in healthcare services, including a shortage of physicians and the absence of health facilities managing stroke, such as stroke units and centers [9, 10]. In a systematic review, it was found that epidemiological studies for stroke in Africa are mostly hospital-based studies and may not represent the actual incidence or prevalence, as patients with minor strokes or rapidly fatal strokes may not get hospitalized [9, 11]. Despite this bias, stroke accounts for 65% of different neurological disorders affecting hospitalized adults in Nigeria [12]. A rise in stroke admissions was reported in Tanzanian hospital-based studies (an increase from 23 to 86 per 100,000 over 27 years) as well as in Ghanaian studies (from 50 to 622 per 100,000 over 33 years) [13]. Such an increase in admission might highlight the increasing burden of stroke, more awareness of stroke, and the demographic shift from rural to urban in many African countries [9, 10, 14]. Other hospital-based studies found incidence ranging from 31 per 100,000 in Zimbabwe to 149 per 100,000 in Mozambique [15, 16]. Community studies in upper Egypt found an incidence of 181 and 250 per 100,000 [17, 18], whilst the incidence was 25 per 100,000 in Nigeria and between 108 and 316 per 100,000 in Tanzania [19, 20].

The prevalence of stroke varies greatly in different countries. The crude prevalence rate was as low as 15 per 100,000 population in rural Ethiopia [21], 42 in Tunisia [22], 114 in Nigeria [23], 243 in South Africa [24], 284 in Morocco [25], 460, and 1156 in two studies in Benin [26, 27], 922 and 963 in upper Egypt [28, 29]; and 1230 and 1460 along the Niger Delta region in Nigeria [30, 31]. The highest prevalence was 2300 per 100,000 population in Tanzania [32].

The incidence and prevalence for all kinds of strokes are on the rise compared to the rest of the world, and this could be explained based on demographic changes as in the case of increased longevity secondary to better control of communicable diseases and shifting in the community from rural to urban with its associated stress, modifiable vascular risk factors as sedentary lifestyle, food rich in carbohydrates and fats with its associated dyslipidemia, hypertension, and diabetes [33, 34]. Moreover, if the study conducted in Tanzania, Hai as a rural area and Dar Es Salaam as an urban area, is generalized, according to Akinyemi et al., then one in six Africans will suffer a stroke every minute [34].

2.3 Burden of stroke in Africa (mortality, and fatality)

Stroke mortality in Africa is one of the highest in the world, ranging between 5.5 and 11% [35–37], and in some studies, the one-month case fatality exceeds 45% and might reach 83.3% [38]. This could be attributed to deficiencies in the proper implementation of stroke services in many African countries. There is a shortage of neurologists, and in many instances, general practitioners or even traditional and complementary medicine practitioners are first line in treating stroke [10, 39]. In addition, other shortfalls include delay in presentation, lack of reperfusion for ischemic stroke or surgical intervention for intracerebral hemorrhage, inadequate management of stroke-related complications such as pneumonia or sepsis, and lack of access to physiotherapy [10, 34].

2.4 Stroke subtype

Globally, rates of ischemic strokes (62.4%) are higher compared to intracerebral hemorrhage (27.9%) and subarachnoid hemorrhage (9.7%) [40]. This is also the case in Africa, including SSA, irrespective of age [9, 41–46]. In the INTERSTROKE study, hemorrhagic strokes accounted for 9% of cases seen in high-income countries (HIC) vs. 34% in African countries [47]. This reflects that a greater burden of hypertension is in Africa since it has been shown that the proportion of hemorrhagic strokes in a population correlates with the burden and severity of uncontrolled hypertension [47, 48].

2.5 Risk factors

Two major studies, INTERSTROKE and Stroke Investigative Research and Educational Network Study (SIREN), assessed stroke risk factors. For INTERSTROKE, it was conducted in Mozambique, Nigeria, South Africa, Sudan, and Uganda; for SIREN, it was conducted in Nigeria and Ghana. Despite the belief that communicable diseases such as HIV might share in a good sum of stroke risks in Africa, the two studies found that modifiable vascular risks are similar to developed world and are pivotal and more important in Africa [49, 50]. The two studies found that hypertension, dyslipidemia, diabetes mellitus, central obesity, cardiac disorders, smoking, an unhealthy diet rich in salt and protein, and poor in fresh leafy vegetables, as well as high alcohol consumption, physical inactivity, and psychosocial stress are all common contributors to stroke [49, 50].

Hypertension was found to be a major contributor risk factor, and this might explain the higher rate of intracerebral hemorrhage in SSA. In Africa, more than 45% of the population above the age of 25 are hypertensives, and around 50% of hypertensives are unaware, undiagnosed, uncontrolled, and uncompliant [51]. Hypertension aggravates atherosclerosis by inducing complex vascular micro-aneurysm formation, lipohyalinosis, and micro atheroma, resulting in rupture or occlusion of the vessel, leading to intracerebral hemorrhage or ischemia, respectively.

Dyslipidemia was the second most common risk factor; meanwhile, and despite being one of the major causes of morbidity and mortality, yet cardiac disease came sixth in risk factors for stroke, with only 7% detected Atrial Fibrillation (AF) in the INTERSTROKE study, which is a much lower percentage for SSA if compared to NA. AF leads to uncoordinated contractions and stasis, most marked at the left atrial appendage [52]. This causes increased concentrations of fibrinogen, D-dimer, and von Willebrand factor, which are indicative of prothrombotic states and dislodgement of thrombus leading to cerebral infarction [52]. AF, coupled with other risk factors such as hypertension, cardiac diseases, tobacco smoking, and sleep apnea, further increases the likelihood of succumbing to a stroke [53]. Diabetes was ranked seventh and eighth for INTERSTROKE and SIREN, respectively [34]. It leads to atherosclerosis either alone or in combination with other atherogenic risk factors such as hypertension, obesity, and dyslipidemia, leading to thrombus formation [54]. Compared to the general population, individuals with diabetes have a fourfold higher risk of stroke.

Factors that affect the vessel wall integrity or the vascular content also play a role in stroke development. HIV is highly prevalent in SSA, with over 25 million adults now living with HIV infection [55]. With expanded access to anti-retroviral therapy (ART), people with HIV are living longer and experiencing fewer opportunistic infections, but conversely are experiencing an emerging rise in cardiovascular diseases, including stroke [55, 56]. HIV increases the risk of stroke through its inflammatory sequel to the endothelium, induced vasculitis, hypercoagulopathy, and the adverse effects of retroviral therapy (vasculopathy, induced dyslipidemia, and insulin resistance) [57, 58].

Rheumatic heart disease is by far the most important form of acquired heart disease in children and young adults in LMIC [59]. The predominant valvular lesion commonly associated with systemic embolization is mitral stenosis, usually observed in the third decade [60]. Mitral stenosis has a 30% risk of systemic thromboembolism leading to stroke, and the risk of recurrence is as high as 60% in the first year [61, 62]. In SSA, where the burden of rheumatic heart disease is high, it is an important risk factor for stroke in young adults that warrants studying [63, 64]. Two-thirds of sickle cell disease (SCD) patients are in Africa; it was found that SCD accounts for 4.2% of strokes in Africa. SCD is responsible for occluding distal circulation within the circle of Willis [65].

Many viral infections and febrile illnesses were reported to take place around 10 days before stroke in many Africans. In Nigeria and Ghana, 10% of stroke victims reported fever up to 4 weeks before stroke development; this highlights an unstudied role of viral infections and fever in stroke [66]. The COVID-19 burden on stroke showed a rising trend in many African countries. In one year since its declaration as a pandemic, 47 African countries reported 7.1 million infections, amounting to 2.5% of the global burden of COVID-19 [67]. COVID-19 affects the endothelium integrity as well as the angiotensin-converting enzyme receptors, with a further rise in the risk of blood pressure as well as coagulopathy, which in turn increases stroke risk directly or indirectly through augmenting risk factors such as uncontrolled blood pressure [68, 69].

2.6 Conclusion

The epidemiology of stroke in Africa needs further in-depth analysis and studies with two major defects, first is in-hospital-based data, which might be deficient in representing the true country stroke status owing to that not all stroke cases are admitted, and of those not admitted and die out of stroke, stroke as a direct cause of death might not be properly stated in the registries, second, and despite that there is some community-based studies yet not covering all African countries.

Risk factors of stroke are nearly similar between different African countries and worldwide, with hypertension being a leading cause, and this might explain the prevalence of haemorrhagic stroke (HS) in SSA. Communicable diseases such as HIV and other forms of febrile viral infections might have some role in stroke development in African countries, and hematologic disorders, precisely SCD, account for a risk in stroke development in Africa compared to other countries worldwide.

3. China

3.1 Background

China is a country with a population of 1.4 billion people and is the second most populous country in the world after India. With rapid economic progress, the average life expectancy has increased from 33 years in 1960 to 79 years in 2022 [70]. With an aging population, stroke remains an important cause of mortality and morbidity.

Prevalence and incidence.

Between 1990 and 2019, the incidence of stroke in China increased by 123% to 276.7 per 100,000 person-years in 2019 [71]. The incidence is greater in the older population, with an estimated 500 per 100,000 person-years in people older than 40 years and as high as 2749 per 100,000 person-years after 80 years [72]. However, when the age of the overall population is considered, the age-standardized incidence rates decreased by 9.3% between 1990 and 2019 [71].

Of the 3.94 million incident strokes in 2019, 2.87 million were ischemic strokes, 0.85 million were intracerebral hemorrhages, and 0.22 million were subarachnoid hemorrhages [71]. The increase in stroke incidence was the highest in ischemic stroke (226.5%), followed by subarachnoid hemorrhage (35.6% and intracerebral hemorrhage (17.6%) [71]. However, age-standardized incidence rates of intracerebral hemorrhage and subarachnoid hemorrhage had decreased, whilst ischemic stroke increased between 1990 and 2019 [71].

The prevalence of stroke was on the rise as well. In 2019, the prevalence of stroke was 28.8 million, a 147% rise from 1990. The increase in prevalence was largest in ischemic stroke (24.8 million, 195% increase) compared to intracerebral hemorrhage (4.4 million, 43% increase) and subarachnoid hemorrhage (1.5 million, 55% increase) [71]. The prevalence rate increased in people ≥60 years but decreased in people <60 years, highlighting the major contribution of aging to the burden of stroke in China [71].

3.2 Outcomes after stroke

Despite an increase in the number of deaths due to stroke and mortality rate since the 1990s, age-standardized mortality had reduced in all subtypes of stroke, with the largest decline in subarachnoid hemorrhage (reduction of 84%) followed by intracerebral hemorrhage (reduction of 48%) and ischemic stroke (reduction of 3%) [71]. This may be due to a gradual but substantial improvement in the quality of stroke care [73, 74]. The prognosis of acute stroke patients appeared to be better compared to HICs, in part due to the younger age of onset and milder stroke [74, 75]. Disability-adjusted life years (DALYs) of stroke have increased steadily since 1990. However, there is a reduction in the age-standardized DALY rate by 42% between 1990 and 2019 [71]. The economic burden of stroke is massive. In 2018, the direct costs of stroke were ¥247.8 billion (purchasing power parity-$PPP 58.6 billion), and the indirect costs were ¥704.4 billion ($PPP 166.5 billion) [76]. As approximately 70% of stroke costs come from public funding, this constitutes a significant economic burden on the Chinese economy [76].

3.3 Risk factors for stroke

Hypertension, dyslipidemia, diabetes mellitus, excessive alcohol intake, air pollution, high salt, and low fruit and vegetable diet are the most common risk factors for stroke [49, 77, 78]. Hypertension is highly prevalent, affecting 28% of the population. Between 2002 and 2014, the number of people with hypertension nearly doubled from 153 million to 300 million [79]. In addition, less than 20% of patients with hypertension had adequate blood pressure control [80].

Dyslipidemia and diabetes mellitus are common, affecting 34% and 11% of the population, respectively, and are poorly controlled [81, 82]. Lifestyle factors put men at higher risk of stroke as well. As high as two-thirds of men are smokers and one-third drink alcohol weekly compared to <5% in women [83, 84].

3.4 Geographical differences

Geographical location was a factor that contributed to the burden of stroke in China [77, 85]. The incidence of stroke was the highest in the northeastern (441–486/100,000 person-years) and the lowest in the southern region (81–136/100,000 person-years) [86]. The higher incidence of stroke may be associated with a higher prevalence of hypertension in the northeastern and northern regions [87]. In addition, there is a higher proportion of smoking and alcohol consumption in the northeast region [77]. Dietary differences contribute to a higher incidence of stroke, where the northern Chinese diet is high in salted vegetables, and the southern Chinese diet is characterized by high intakes of vegetables and fruits and lower salt intake [88].

Rural areas had a higher incidence and prevalence of stroke due to differences in prevalence of risk factors and their treatment [77, 85, 89, 90]. The awareness, treatment, and control of hypertension, diabetes mellitus, and dyslipidemia are less optimal in the rural areas [79, 81, 82, 87]. Smoking prevalence is higher, whilst consumption of vegetables and fruits is lower in rural areas [91]. In addition, the common domestic use of coal and wood as fuels in rural areas contributes to the release of fine particulate matter (PM) and increases the risk of stroke mortality [92].

3.5 Conclusions

Due to an aging population, the overall incidence and prevalence of stroke have been on the rise. Hypertension is a major risk factor for stroke and is poorly controlled. There are vast geographical differences in the burden of stroke and its risk factors between different regions and rural–urban differences. These factors should be considered with planning health policies to reduce the stroke burden.

4. Europe

4.1 Background

Europe has a population of 742 million as of 2023, having diverse demographic trends across its regions. The European Union (EU), comprising 27 member states, has a population of 448 million people. Europe's median age is among the highest globally, with 21% of the population being aged 65 and over, and a life expectancy of 81.5 years in 2023, with important variations between regions and countries. Eastern European countries, most of them being considered low- to middle-income countries, present distinct demographic characteristics influenced by their socioeconomic and historical factors, marked by demographic decline, high level of emigration, and lower life expectancy when compared with Western Europe [93]. The health care systems of this region exhibit notable differences, with funding and access to services being higher in Western countries, infrastructure and health education levels in the population being lower in Eastern European countries when compared to Western countries. According to the World Bank, globally there are 132 countries classified as low- or middle-income countries (LMICs), seven LMICs being from Europe, most of them from Eastern and Southern Europe [5].

4.2 Burden of stroke

Eastern Europe recorded the highest number of stroke cases, followed by Western and Central Europe. Between 2010 and 2019, the incidence rates remained stable across all these subregions; however, age-standardized incidence rates showed a consistent decline in all the subregions, except for the individuals from Eastern and Central Europe below 70 years, where rates remained unchanged. Eastern Europe had the highest age-standardized incidence rate, 2.75 times greater than in Western Europe, despite a significant reduction in incidence rates across all subregions over the past decades. The total number of prevalent stroke cases rose by 4%, reaching more than 14 million cases between 2010 and 2019. Ischemic stroke accounted for 78.9%, while intracerebral hemorrhages and subarachnoid hemorrhages made up 14.4% and 10.6%, respectively.

When examining all the regions in Europe, the absolute number of stroke cases increased in Western and Central Europe but remained stable in Eastern Europe. Overall age-standardized prevalence rates declined across all subregions. However, there was an approximately 4% rise in age-standardized prevalence among individuals under 70 in Eastern and Central Europe. Eastern Europe had the highest age-standardized prevalence rate, which was 1.8 times greater than in Western Europe. Regarding stroke-related deaths, the absolute number increased significantly in Western Europe, while remaining stable in Eastern Europe, but still at a higher level compared to the other regions. Although, Eastern Europe had the highest age-adjusted mortality rate, it also experienced the most significant decline in mortality rates between 2010 and 2019, with a decrease of more than 20%, this improvement being caused mainly by better health policies, higher levels of investments and better quality of care [94, 95].

The total disability-adjusted life years lost (DALYs) rates have been declining across Europe, in both genders, over the timespan of 30 years, between 1990 and 2019, with the Eastern European region experiencing the highest burden of disease from ischemic and hemorrhagic (intracerebral and subarachnoid hemorrhage (SAH)) stroke, followed by Central Europe. In 1990, DALY rates for the female gender were approximately identical in Eastern Europe and Central Europe and higher by 25–26% than in Western Europe. As the years passed, Central Europe observed the highest reduction of stroke burden in women, reducing the gap with Western Europe to 9%, while Eastern Europe experienced an increase from 26–32% in 2019. The burden of disease is greater in men (with a male–female ratio of 1.3 in Western Europe and 1.5 in Eastern Europe in 2019) and the difference in stroke burden across regions is also higher in the male population, with Eastern Europe having the lowest decline in stroke incidence and DALYs, by 16% from 1990 to 2019.

All the countries in Central and Eastern Europe experienced a decline in disease burden [96], although they had different trends and patterns. The smallest decrease was observed in LMICs like Montenegro (−5%), North Macedonia (−16%), Bosnia and Herzegovina (−19%), and Albania (−28%), with North Macedonia having the highest health loss due to stroke in 2019, which is 7.7 times higher than the rates in Western Europe. There is a substantial variation in stroke burden between the countries from the Central and Eastern European regions. The variation was larger among the Central European countries, and it was driven mainly by the very high stroke burden rates of three Balkan countries, those being North Macedonia, Montenegro, and Serbia. A possible explanation for this may be related to the fact that the highest rates of years of life lost (YLLs) due to stroke are found in North Macedonia, Montenegro, and Serbia, suggesting differences in the quality of acute stroke care in those countries compared to the rest of Central Europe.

4.3 Stroke subtypes

There are differences reported about the relative proportions of each stroke based on pathophysiological subtypes in various regions and countries of Europe, as previously reported on a global scale [97]. There were countries where the proportion of total stroke burden due to intracerebral hemorrhage reached 75% in Montenegro and 71% in Albania among men in 2019. Among Eastern European countries, Moldova had a higher proportion of stroke burden due to intracerebral hemorrhage, which may be related to greater total stroke burden due to YLLs in these countries (up to 90%). While the proportion of total stroke burden from SAH did not vary as much as for the other pathological subtypes, the lack of access to treatments for ruptured cerebral aneurysms and the sequelae of SAH likely contributes to a disproportionate burden of YLLs in Eastern and Central Europe.

5. India

5.1 Burden of stroke

India is the most populous country in the world, with a population of 1.45 billion people [98]. Life expectancy in India has increased beyond 60 years of age, which has led to a progressive increase in noncommunicable age-related disorders [99, 100]. Stroke burden is increasing in India, and it is the fourth leading cause of death and the fifth leading cause of disability in the country [101]. The Indian Global Burden of Disease Study 1990–2019 estimated stroke to be the largest contributor to disability-adjusted life years (DALYs) with an approximate contribution of 37.9% [102]. The incidence of stroke in India is between 105 and 152/100,000 people per year [103], and the age and sex-standardized mortality rate is 82.4 per 100,000 person-years [104]. The one-month fatality from stroke ranges between 18 and 42% (4), which is much higher than in developed nations.

A recent systematic review by Jones et al. [101] found that the median age of stroke patients in India was 62.2 years, with a male preponderance (59%), with a higher stroke incidence in men. Lower female representation could likely be due to gender discrimination in access to healthcare, with studies revealing that it was worse for women, with a male-to-female sex ratio of 1.69 for outpatient visits [105]. The mean age for stroke occurrence was lower in Indian patients compared to the global average [106]. Approximately 20% of first-ever stroke patients admitted were found to be younger than 40 years of age. The annual stroke incidence in individuals between 18 and 49 years was found to be 46 per 100,000 person-years [107], which was significantly greater than the European (5–15 per 100,000) and American population (20 per 100,000) [108]. Strokes in this economically productive age group lead to multiple social, emotional, economic, vocational, and physical considerations [109].

Although the one-month case fatality rate ranged between 18 and 42%, higher death rates were found in men compared to women. Also, the Million Death Study [110] found that approximately 33% of premature stroke deaths were reported from the Eastern part of the country which could be attributable to ethnic differences (higher rates of hypertension and dietary habits of increased salt intake).

5.2 Stroke subtypes

The rates of ischemic stroke varied between 65 and 84%, with large artery and small vessel stroke subtypes being more common than cardioembolic ones [104]. This could, in part, be due to the greater prevalence of intracranial atherosclerotic disease among Asian (and Indian) stroke patients [111]. Among other determined etiologies, stroke due to infectious diseases, although uncommon, was more common than elsewhere, with tuberculosis, fungal infections, and infective endocarditis being the leading culprits [111]. Tuberculosis causes stroke involving the basal ganglia secondary to tubercular meningitis associated with basal arachnoiditis around the circle of Willis. Thrombocytopenia with viral infections like dengue has occasionally led to intracerebral hemorrhage (ICH) [112]. The rate of ICH was found to be between 20 and 32% [104], which is higher than in Western countries. Overall, the rate of ICH was found to be the highest in Asia among all continents [113].

Although cerebral venous sinus thrombosis (CVT) [114] is an uncommon cause of stroke in India, it was found to affect predominantly young people (median age—31 years) and is more prevalent during the summer months [114, 115]. The risk factors mostly identified were anemia, oral contraceptives, pregnancy, puerperium, and central nervous system (CNS) infections [115]. Another study found that among pregnant CVT patients, 34% had more than one CVT-predisposing prothrombotic factor [116].

5.3 Conclusion

High-quality epidemiological stroke data from India is heterogeneous and incomplete since it is only representative of four out of the 29 states and seven union territories of the country. To further identify the stroke burden in India, future, more detailed studies following the WHO STEPS framework [117] would be required.

6. South America and the Caribbean

6.1 Background

Stroke is a leading cause of morbidity and mortality in Latin America and the Caribbean (LAC). With a population exceeding 666 million [118] (World Meter, 2025), the region's socioeconomic, cultural, and geographic diversity results in significant variations in stroke incidence, prevalence, etiology, risk factors, healthcare, and outcomes. Stroke poses a major public health challenge due to its high burden on healthcare systems and its impact on individuals and families [119].

6.2 Incidence and mortality rates

Stroke epidemiology in LAC is characterized by considerable regional variability, with stroke incidence rates differing widely across countries. A pooled analysis of data from multiple studies indicated an overall incidence of 255 stroke cases per 100,000 person-years in South America, with men exhibiting higher rates (261 per 100,000) compared to women (217 per 100,000) [120]. This regional variability in stroke incidence reflects differences in healthcare infrastructure, socioeconomic status, and the prevalence of risk factors.

Data from a systematic review spanning from 1997 to 2021 reported an annual stroke incidence of 119 cases per 100,000 individuals across LAC, with a prevalence of 3060 cases per 100,000 individuals [121]. In contrast, earlier population-based studies have shown that stroke incidence varied from 0.35 to 1.83 per 1000 individuals annually, while prevalence ranged between 1.74 and 6.51 per 1000 individuals [122].

This variation underscores the changing landscape of stroke epidemiology in the region, with differences in data collection methods and healthcare access contributing to evolving figures.

In 2019, LAC accounted for the fourth largest stroke burden globally, with 6.8 million disability-adjusted life years (DALYs). The majority of this burden was attributed to premature deaths (89.5% of DALYs), and intracerebral hemorrhage emerged as the leading cause of overall stroke burden, responsible for 42% of DALYs. Ischemic stroke, on the other hand, was the leading cause of disability, contributing to 69% of years lived with disability [123].

6.3 Younger people

Several studies have identified an unfavorable temporal trend in stroke incidence among younger people in LAC, particularly among young women. While the global incidence of stroke declined in older people between 2010 and 2019, a similar trend was not observed in younger people in LAC. Instead, the incidence of stroke has risen. This has been linked to increasing rates of conventional risk factors, such as arterial hypertension, obesity, physical inactivity, dyslipidemia, diabetes mellitus, and smoking, alongside emerging factors like air pollution, long working hours, and stress. Moreover, better access to acute stroke care and improved patient awareness have also contributed to the rising numbers [124].

6.4 Risk factors and population-attributable fractions

The high burden of stroke in LAC can largely be attributed to modifiable risk factors. Arterial hypertension remains the most significant contributor to stroke risk in the region, responsible for approximately 53% of the population-attributable fraction [123]. Obesity is another key risk factor, contributing to 37% of stroke cases. These risk factors are particularly influential in hemorrhagic strokes, which disproportionately affect women and older adults [123].

In lower-income countries within LAC, household air pollution is emerging as a critical risk factor, further complicating the stroke epidemiology in these settings. The higher prevalence of metabolic conditions, including high blood pressure and elevated body mass index, combined with limited access to prevention and treatment, particularly in rural areas, exacerbates the stroke burden in these nations [122, 123].

6.5 Case fatality and mortality trends

The case-fatality rate for stroke in LAC remains alarmingly high, with studies indicating rates ranging from 20 to 40% depending on the country. In particular, the 30-day case-fatality rate following a first stroke was reported as 21.1% in recent analyses. The high mortality rates are compounded by limited access to specialized acute stroke care, including thrombolysis and mechanical thrombectomy, and also by a lack of sufficient post-stroke rehabilitation, especially in lower-resource settings [119, 121, 125].

6.6 Economic impact and cost of stroke care

The financial burden of stroke treatment is another critical issue in LAC. A multicenter study assessed the direct costs associated with acute ischemic stroke treatment in various LAC countries [126]. The analysis revealed significant cost disparities, with costs ranging from I$ 5902 in Peru to I$ 27,488 in Brazil for the same treatment. The study further highlighted the variations in costs for different treatment modalities, including medical treatment, intravenous thrombolysis, mechanical thrombectomy, and the combination of both, with costs ranging from I$ 9735 to I$ 30,153 depending on the treatment approach. These cost differences reflect the diversity in healthcare systems, access to treatment, and regional disparities in economic resources. Addressing these disparities through targeted interventions, improving access to care, and optimizing healthcare spending are essential to improving stroke outcomes across LAC [126].

6.7 Conclusion

Stroke continues to impose a significant burden on public health in Latin America and the Caribbean, with increasing incidence rates, high mortality and case-fatality rates, and substantial regional disparities in care. The rising prevalence of risk factors such as arterial hypertension, obesity, and diabetes mellitus, compounded by emerging environmental risks, calls for urgent public health action. Furthermore, disparities in access to care and the economic burden of stroke treatment must be addressed through more equitable healthcare policies, better prevention strategies, and efficient allocation of resources.

Improving stroke outcomes in LAC will require comprehensive approaches that target modifiable risk factors, enhance stroke care infrastructure, and ensure more equitable access to treatment, especially in underserved areas. As stroke epidemiology continues to evolve, ongoing research and collaboration will be crucial to developing effective strategies for reducing the stroke burden in this diverse and rapidly changing region.

7. Southeast Asia

7.1 Background

Southeast Asia (SEA) represents a diverse sub-region of Asia, encompassing 11 nations: Brunei, Cambodia, Indonesia, Laos, Malaysia, Myanmar, Philippines, Singapore, Thailand, Timor-Leste, and Vietnam. The region spans approximately 4.5 million square kilometers and hosts a population exceeding 680 million, making it one of the world's most densely populated regions [4]. Population projections indicate continued growth, with expectations of reaching 760 million by 2050, driven by high birth rates and improving life expectancy [127].

The region exhibits remarkable cultural, ethnic, and linguistic diversity, predominantly composed of Austronesian, Austroasiatic, Tai-Kadai, and Sino-Tibetan ethnic groups. The religious landscape is equally varied, with Islam, Buddhism, Christianity, and Hinduism serving as major faiths. Economically, SEA presents a spectrum ranging from low-income countries to upper-middle-income nations, with Singapore standing as the region's sole high-income country [127].

7.2 Epidemiological patterns and disease burden

The Global Burden of Disease Study 2019 revealed that stroke remains the second leading cause of death in Southeast Asia, with low-income countries experiencing a significantly higher burden than high-income nations [128]. Specifically, World Bank low-income countries faced 3.6 times higher age-standardized stroke mortality rates (95% CI: 3.5–3.8) and 3.7 times higher disability-adjusted life year (DALY) rates (95% CI: 3.5–3.9), exceeding the global average of 11.6% [128]. The disparity is further emphasized by the fact that 86.0% (85.9–86.9) of all stroke-related deaths and 89.0% (88.9–89.3) of stroke-related DALYs occurred in lower-income, lower-middle-income, and upper-middle-income countries [128]. A comprehensive WHO report published in 2021 highlights that the burden is particularly significant in low- and middle-income countries, which account for over 85% of global stroke mortality [129].

Southeast Asian countries show significant variations in stroke burden, with Indonesia demonstrating the highest mortality rate of 193.3 per 100,000 person-years, followed by Myanmar (165.4), Lao PDR (141.3), and Cambodia (137.8). The middle-range countries include the Philippines (109.6) and Vietnam (124.5), while Malaysia shows a lower rate at 84.3 per 100,000 person-years [7]. The lowest mortality rates are observed in Singapore (47.9), Thailand (62.8), and Brunei (68.6) per 100,000 person-years. Regarding stroke incidence, limited data are available for Southeast Asian countries, with Malaysia reporting the lowest rate at 67 per 100,000 person-years, Vietnam at 250 per 100,000 person-years, and Singapore at 180 per 100,000 person-years [104]. When examining DALYs lost, a similar pattern emerges with Indonesia showing the highest burden, followed by Myanmar, Lao PDR, and Cambodia, while Singapore demonstrates the lowest burden in the region [104].

7.3 Young stroke

The burden of stroke among young adults (aged ≤50 years) has emerged as a significant public health challenge in Southeast Asia, with epidemiological data indicating substantially higher prevalence rates compared to Western populations [128]. This concerning trend is attributed to a complex interplay of modifiable risk factors, including increasing prevalence of hypertension and diabetes mellitus at younger ages, rapid urbanization-associated lifestyle changes, and region-specific genetic predispositions. Recent epidemiological surveillance data demonstrate that Southeast Asia bears a disproportionate burden of young stroke, with urbanization and socioeconomic transitions driving significant shifts in dietary patterns and physical activity levels [5]. Moreover, the healthcare infrastructure challenges, particularly in resource-limited settings, contribute to delayed diagnosis and suboptimal risk factor management [5]. These findings underscore the urgent need for targeted public health interventions, emphasizing primary prevention strategies and early risk factor modification, to address this emerging epidemic in the region.

7.4 Cerebrovascular disease patterns

Intracranial arterial stenosis (ICAS) patterns in Southeast Asia demonstrate distinct characteristics. Hospital-based studies from Southeast Asian countries show varying distributions, with Indonesia reporting high rates of large artery atherosclerosis at 59.6% [130], while Singapore shows a predominance of small vessel disease at 47.9% [131]. Traditional cardiovascular risk factors remain consistent with other Asian regions, though the impact may vary across different Southeast Asian populations.

7.5 Distinctive vascular conditions

While Moyamoya disease (MMD) is less commonly reported in Southeast Asia compared to East Asia, other vascular conditions show regional significance. Studies from Thailand have documented cases of cerebral gnathostomiasis, a parasitic infestation unique to the region that can cause subarachnoid hemorrhage and migratory intracerebral hemorrhage [132]. The pattern of arterial dissections in Southeast Asian populations remains understudied compared to East Asian cohorts.

7.6 Infection-related cerebrovascular complications

Southeast Asia faces unique challenges from tropical infectious diseases affecting cerebrovascular health. Dengue hemorrhagic fever, prevalent in the region, can result in intracranial hemorrhage due to thrombocytopenia [133]. Recent studies have also highlighted the impact of COVID-19 on stroke presentations in Southeast Asian healthcare systems [134].

7.7 Less common vascular conditions

In Southeast Asia, radiation vasculopathy presents a significant clinical challenge, particularly due to the high prevalence of nasopharyngeal carcinoma (NPC) in the region [135]. Studies from Southeast Asian centers, particularly in Singapore and Malaysia, have reported favorable experiences with carotid artery stenting (CAS) for radiation-induced carotid artery stenosis [136]. A meta-analysis demonstrated that NPC patients treated with radiation therapy had an increased risk of carotid stenosis, with a relative risk of 4.17 ($p < 0.00001$) compared to non-irradiated patients [137]. Regional institutions have adopted surveillance strategies using carotid ultrasound screening one year after radiation therapy, with close monitoring for disease progression.

7.8 Future directions

The challenges in Southeast Asian stroke care require targeted interventions focusing on strengthening primary prevention, particularly for young stroke patients. Key priorities include developing telemedicine networks to bridge urban–rural divides, training more stroke specialists, and establishing more acute stroke units in underserved areas. Healthcare financing reforms are needed to reduce out-of-pocket expenses for acute stroke treatments, while regional collaboration could optimize resource utilization and improve access to advanced therapies.

7.9 Conclusion

Southeast Asia faces unique challenges in stroke care, marked by significant healthcare disparities across countries and a concerning trend of increasing young stroke incidence. While some nations have established comprehensive stroke systems, many struggle with limited resources and healthcare access. Success in addressing these challenges will require a sustained commitment to improving infrastructure, increasing specialized workforce capacity, and implementing targeted public health interventions that consider the region's socioeconomic diversity and unique disease patterns.

8. COVID-19 and stroke

COVID-19 significantly impacted stroke care worldwide, but its effects have been especially severe in LMICs, where healthcare systems were already under strain.

The pathophysiology of stroke in COVID-19 patients is multifactorial and complex, involving both direct and indirect effects of the virus on the vascular and nervous systems. SARS-CoV-2, the virus responsible for COVID-19, binds to angiotensin-converting enzyme 2 (ACE2) receptors, which are expressed in endothelial cells, neurons, and glial tissue. This interaction can trigger widespread endothelial dysfunction and inflammation, leading to a prothrombotic state. The exaggerated immune response, or "cytokine storm," seen in severe cases, leads to elevated levels of inflammatory markers like IL-6 and C-reactive protein (CRP), further promoting coagulation and platelet activation. Additionally, COVID-19 is associated with increased levels of D-dimer and fibrinogen, indicating hypercoagulability and increased risk of thromboembolic events, including large vessel occlusion strokes. Cardiac complications such as arrhythmias and myocarditis may also increase the risk of cardioembolic strokes. In some cases, autoimmune mechanisms and antiphospholipid antibodies may also play a role. Together, these factors contribute to an increased incidence of ischemic stroke, particularly in younger patients without traditional risk factors, underlining the need for vigilance and early intervention in COVID-19-associated stroke [138–140].

However, in LMICs, limited access to diagnostic tools, delayed hospital presentations, and shortages of trained personnel often hinder timely diagnosis and treatment [141]. Lockdowns and fear of infection further discouraged patients from seeking urgent care, leading to a rise in untreated or late-presenting strokes. Telemedicine, which offered a lifeline in high-income settings, remained inaccessible to many in LMICs due to technological and infrastructural barriers. Moreover, many of the existing stroke units were reallocated to manage the pandemic, and this further compromised the stroke care. As a result, mortality and disability from stroke increased disproportionately in these regions.

Addressing this crisis requires targeted strategies, such as strengthening stroke care pathways, investing in public awareness, and ensuring equitable access to acute stroke interventions, even during pandemics. The COVID-19 experience highlights the urgent need to build resilient stroke systems in LMICs that can withstand future global health emergencies.

9. Summary of stroke in low- and middle-income countries

Stroke poses a significant and growing public health challenge in low- and middle-income countries (LMICs), where rising incidence rates are fueled by urbanization, sedentary lifestyles, and diets high in salt and fat. Hypertension, diabetes, and limited awareness of risk factors contribute to the burden, compounded by inadequate healthcare infrastructure for timely diagnosis, acute treatment, and rehabilitation. LMICs face higher stroke-related mortality and disability rates compared to high-income nations, as limited access to specialized care, costly therapies, and scarce rehabilitation services exacerbate outcomes. Economic strains on families due to medical expenses and lost income further deepen the crisis. Addressing this requires targeted investments in preventive measures, affordable management of chronic conditions, and strengthening healthcare systems to improve acute care and long-term support for survivors.

Conflict of interest

The authors declare no conflict of interest.

Author details

Zhe Kang Law[1]*, Sarah Shali Matuja[2], Mirjam R. Heldner[3], Tamer Roushdy[4], Ayush Agarwal[5], Maria Khan[6], Bogdan Ciopleias[7], Abdul Hanif Khan Yusof Khan[8] and Selam Kifelew[9]

1 Department of Medicine, Faculty of Medicine, National University of Malaysia, Kuala Lumpur, Malaysia

2 Department of Internal Medicine, Catholic University of Health and Allied Sciences Weill Bugando Mwanza, Tanzania

3 Department of Neurology, Inselspital, University Hospital and University of Bern, Bern, Switzerland

4 Department of Neurology, Faculty of Medicine, Ain Shams University, Cairo, Egypt

5 Department of Neurology, All India Institute of Medical Sciences, New Delhi, India

6 Department of Neurology Rashid Hospital, Mohammed bin Rashid University of Health Sciences, Dubai, United Arab Emirates

7 Department of Neurology, Faculty of Medicine, Transilvania University Brasov, Romania

8 Department of Neurology, Faculty of Medicine and Health Sciences, Universiti Putra Malaysia, Serdang, Malaysia

9 Department of Neurology, Addis Ababa University, College of Health Sciences, Ethiopia

*Address all correspondence to: zhe.kanglaw@hctm.ukm.edu.my

References

[1] World Health Organisation. The top 10 causes of death. 2024. Available from https://www.who.int/news-room/fact-sheets/detail/the-top-10-causes-of-death [Accessed: December 13, 2024]

[2] Feigin VL, Brainin M, Norrving B, Martins SO, Pandian J, Lindsay P, et al. World stroke organization: Global stroke fact sheet 2025. International Journal of Stroke. 2025;**20**:132-144

[3] GBD 2016 Stroke Collaborators. Global, regional, and national burden of stroke, 1990-2016: A systematic analysis for the Global Burden of Disease Study 2016. Lancet Neurology. 2019;**18**:439-458

[4] United Nations. World population prospects 2024: Summary of results. In: UN DESA/POP/2024/TR/NO. 9. New York: United Nations; 2024

[5] Eric Metreau, Kathryn Elizabeth Young, Shwetha Grace Eapen. World Bank country classification by income level for 2024-2025. 2024. Available from https://blogs.worldbank.org/en/opendata/world-bank-country-classifications-by-income-level-for-2024-2025 [Accessed: December 13, 2024]

[6] Tishkoff SA, Reed FA, Friedlaender FR, Ehret C, Ranciaro A, Froment A, et al. The genetic structure and history of Africans and African Americans. Science. 2009;**324**:1035-1044

[7] Schlebusch CM, Jakobsson M. Tales of human migration, admixture, and selection in Africa. Annual Review of Genomics and Human Genetics. 2018;**19**:405-428

[8] Owolabi MO, Mensah GA, Kimmel PL, Adu D, Ramsay M, Waddy SP, et al. Understanding the rise in cardiovascular diseases in Africa: Harmonising H3Africa genomic epidemiological teams and tools. Cardiovascular Journal of Africa. 2014;**25**:134-136

[9] Owolabi MO, Akarolo-Anthony S, Akinyemi R, Arnett D, Gebregziabher M, Jenkins C, et al. The burden of stroke in Africa: A glance at the present and a glimpse into the future. Cardiovascular Journal of Africa. 2015;**26**:S27-S38

[10] Roushdy T, Aref H, Kesraoui S, Temgoua M, Nono KP, Gebrewold MA, et al. Stroke services in Africa: What is there and what is needed. International Journal of Stroke. 2022;**17**:972-982

[11] Owolabi MO. Taming the burgeoning stroke epidemic in Africa: Stroke quadrangle to the rescue. The West Indian Medical Journal. 2011;**60**:412-421

[12] Ekenze OS, Onwuekwe IO, Ezeala Adikaibe BA. Profile of neurological admissions at the university of Nigeria teaching hospital Enugu. Nigerian Journal of Medicine. 2010;**19**:419-422

[13] Connor MD, Thorogood M, Modi G, Warlow CP. The burden of stroke in sub-Saharan Africa. American Journal of Preventive Medicine. 2007;**33**:172-173

[14] Thomas GS, Wann LS, Allam AH, Thompson RC, Michalik DE, Sutherland ML, et al. Why did ancient people have atherosclerosis?: From autopsies to computed tomography to potential causes. Global Heart. 2014;**9**:229-237

[15] Matenga J, Kitai I, Levy L. Strokes among black people in Harare, Zimbabwe: Results of computed

tomography and associated risk factors. British Medical Journal Clinical Research. 1986;**292**:1649-1651

[16] Damasceno A, Gomes J, Azevedo A, Carrilho C, Lobo V, Lopes H, et al. An epidemiological study of stroke hospitalizations in Maputo, Mozambique: A high burden of disease in a resource-poor country. Stroke. 2010;**41**:2463-2469

[17] Tallawy HN, Farghaly WM, Rageh TA, Shehata GA, Badry R, Metwally NA, et al. Door-to-door survey of major neurological disorders (project) in Al Quseir City, Red Sea governorate, Egypt. Neuropsychiatric Disease and Treatment. 2013;**9**:767-771

[18] Farghaly WM, El-Tallawy HN, Shehata GA, Rageh TA, Abdel-Hakeem NM, Elhamed MA, et al. Epidemiology of nonfatal stroke and transient ischemic attack in Al-Kharga District, New Valley, Egypt. Neuropsychiatric Disease and Treatment. 2013;**9**:1785-1790

[19] Danesi MA, Okubadejo NU, Ojini FI, Ojo OO. Incidence and 30-day case fatality rate of first-ever stroke in urban Nigeria: The prospective community based epidemiology of stroke in Lagos (EPISIL) phase II results. Journal of the Neurological Sciences. 2013;**331**:43-47

[20] Walker R, Whiting D, Unwin N, Mugusi F, Swai M, Aris E, et al. Stroke incidence in rural and urban Tanzania: A prospective, community-based study. Lancet Neurology. 2010;**9**:786-792

[21] Tekle-Haimanot R, Abebe M, Gebre-Mariam A, Forsgren L, Heijbel J, Holmgren G, et al. Community-based study of neurological disorders in rural Central Ethiopia. Neuroepidemiology. 1990;**9**:263-277

[22] Attia Romdhane N, Ben Hamida M, Mrabet A, Larnaout A, Samoud S, Ben Hamda A, et al. Prevalence study of neurologic disorders in Kelibia (Tunisia). Neuroepidemiology. 1993;**12**:285-299

[23] Danesi M, Okubadejo N, Ojini F. Prevalence of stroke in an urban, mixed-income community in Lagos, Nigeria. Neuroepidemiology. 2007;**28**:216-223

[24] Connor MD, Thorogood M, Casserly B, Dobson C, Warlow CP. Prevalence of stroke survivors in rural South Africa: Results from the Southern Africa stroke prevention initiative (SASPI) Agincourt field site. Stroke. 2004;**35**:627-632

[25] Engels T, Baglione Q, Audibert M, Viallefont A, Mourji F, El Alaoui Faris M. Socioeconomic status and stroke prevalence in Morocco: Results from the Rabat-Casablanca study. PLoS One. 2014;**9**:e89271

[26] Cossi MJ, Gobron C, Preux PM, Niama D, Chabriat H, Houinato D. Stroke: Prevalence and disability in Cotonou, Benin. Cerebrovascular Diseases. 2012;**33**:166-172

[27] Adoukonou T, Yahouédéou B, Agbétou M, Hountada H, Choki B, Kossi O, et al. Prevalence of stroke survivors in Parakou in Northern Benin: A door-to-door community survey. Revue Neurologique (Paris). 2020;**176**:839-845

[28] Khedr EM, Elfetoh NA, Al Attar G, Ahmed MA, Ali AM, Hamdy A, et al. Epidemiological study and risk factors of stroke in Assiut governorate, Egypt: Community-based study. Neuroepidemiology. 2013;**40**:288-294

[29] Khedr EM, Fawi G, Abdela M, Mohammed TA, Ahmed MA, El-Fetoh NA, et al. Prevalence of

ischemic and hemorrhagic strokes in Qena governorate, Egypt: Community-based study. Journal of Stroke and Cerebrovascular Diseases. 2014;**23**:1843-1848

[30] Ezejimofor MC, Uthman OA, Maduka O, Ezeabasili AC, Onwuchekwa AC, Ezejimofor BC, et al. Stroke survivors in Nigeria: A door-to-door prevalence survey from the Niger Delta region. Journal of the Neurological Sciences. 2017;**372**:262-269

[31] Onwuchekwa AC, Tobin-West C, Babatunde S. Prevalence and risk factors for stroke in an adult population in a rural community in the Niger Delta, south-South Nigeria. Journal of Stroke and Cerebrovascular Diseases. 2014;**23**:505-510

[32] Dewhurst F, Dewhurst MJ, Gray WK, Aris E, Orega G, Howlett W, et al. The prevalence of neurological disorders in older people in Tanzania. Acta Neurologica Scandinavica. 2013;**127**:198-207

[33] El Nahas NM, Shokri HM, Roushdy TM, Aref HM, Hamed SM, Shalash AS, et al. Urban versus rural Egypt: Stroke risk factors and clinical profile: Cross-sectional observational study. Journal of Stroke and Cerebrovascular Diseases. 2019;**28**:104316

[34] Akinyemi RO, Ovbiagele B, Adeniji OA, Sarfo FS, Abd-Allah F, Adoukonou T, et al. Stroke in Africa: Profile, progress, prospects and priorities. Nature Reviews. Neurology. 2021;**17**:634-656

[35] Obiako OR, Oparah S, Ogunniyi A. Causes of medical coma in adult patients at the university college hospital, Ibadan Nigeria. The Nigerian Postgraduate Medical Journal. 2011;**18**:1-7

[36] Walker RW, Jusabani A, Aris E, Gray WK, Whiting D, Kabadi G, et al. Post-stroke case fatality within an incident population in rural Tanzania. Journal of Neurology, Neurosurgery, and Psychiatry. 2011;**82**:1001-1005

[37] Maredza M, Bertram MY, Tollman SM. Disease burden of stroke in rural South Africa: An estimate of incidence, mortality and disability adjusted life years. BMC Neurology. 2015;**15**:54

[38] Adoukonou T, Kossi O, Fotso Mefo P, Agbétou M, Magne J, Gbaguidi G, et al. Stroke case fatality in sub-Saharan Africa: Systematic review and meta-analysis. International Journal of Stroke. 2021;**16**:902-916

[39] Roushdy T, Alet MJ, Lotlikar R, Ramage E, Ullberg T, Mosconi MG, et al. Applying the world stroke organization roadmap in planning a model for stroke service implementation in Matrouh governorate-Egypt: A world stroke organization young future stroke leaders' analytical study. The Egyptian Journal of Neurology, Psychiatry and Neurosurgery. 2023;**59**:150

[40] Roth GA, Mensah GA, Johnson CO, Addolorato G, Ammirati E, Baddour LM, et al. Global burden of cardiovascular diseases and risk factors, 1990-2019: Update from the GBD 2019 study. Journal of the American College of Cardiology. 2020;**76**:2982-3021

[41] Chraa M, Louhab N, Kissani N. Stroke in young adults: About 128 cases. The Pan African Medical Journal. 2014;**17**:37

[42] Hsu RT, Ardron ME, Brooks W, Cherry D, Taub NA, Botha JL. The 1996 leicestershire community stroke & ethnicity study: Differences and similarities between South Asian and

white strokes. International Journal of Epidemiology. 1999;**28**:853-858

[43] Miah MNA, Azhar MA, Rahman A, Halder D, Akteruzzaman M, Kundu NC. Risk factors of stroke in Young and old age group - A comparative study. Journal of Medicine. 2012;**13**:138-142

[44] Onwuchekwa AC, Onwuchekwa RC, Asekomeh EG. Stroke in young Nigerian adults. Journal of Vascular Nursing. 2009;**27**:98-102

[45] Owolabi MO, Ugoya S, Platz T. Racial disparity in stroke risk factors: The Berlin-Ibadan experience; a retrospective study. Acta Neurologica Scandinavica. 2009;**119**:81-87

[46] Walker RW, Jusabani A, Aris E, Gray WK, Mitra D, Swai M. A prospective study of stroke sub-type from within an incident population in Tanzania. South African Medical Journal. 2011;**101**:338-344

[47] O'Donnell MJ, Xavier D, Liu L, Zhang H, Chin SL, Rao-Melacini P, et al. Risk factors for ischaemic and intracerebral haemorrhagic stroke in 22 countries (the INTERSTROKE study): A case-control study. Lancet. 2010;**376**:112-123

[48] Namale G, Kamacooko O, Kinengyere A, Yperzeele L, Cras P, Ddumba E, et al. Risk factors for hemorrhagic and ischemic stroke in sub-Saharan Africa. Journal of Tropical Medicine. 2018;**2018**:4650851

[49] O'Donnell MJ, Chin SL, Rangarajan S, Xavier D, Liu L, Zhang H, et al. Global and regional effects of potentially modifiable risk factors associated with acute stroke in 32 countries (INTERSTROKE): A case-control study. Lancet. 2016;**388**:761-775

[50] Owolabi MO, Sarfo F, Akinyemi R, Gebregziabher M, Akpa O, Akpalu A, et al. Dominant modifiable risk factors for stroke in Ghana and Nigeria (SIREN): A case-control study. The Lancet Global Health. 2018;**6**:e436-e446

[51] Geldsetzer P, Manne-Goehler J, Marcus ME, Ebert C, Zhumadilov Z, Wesseh CS, et al. The state of hypertension care in 44 low-income and middle-income countries: A cross-sectional study of nationally representative individual-level data from 1·1 million adults. Lancet. 2019;**394**:652-662

[52] Arboix A, Alió J. Cardioembolic stroke: Clinical features, specific cardiac disorders and prognosis. Current Cardiology Reviews. 2010;**6**:150-161

[53] Kamel H, Okin PM, Elkind MS, Iadecola C. Atrial fibrillation and mechanisms of stroke: Time for a new model. Stroke. 2016;**47**:895-900

[54] Dutton GR, Lewis CE. The look AHEAD trial: Implications for lifestyle intervention in type 2 diabetes mellitus. Progress in Cardiovascular Diseases. 2015;**58**:69-75

[55] UNAIDS. In Danger: UNAIDS Global AIDS Update 2022. 2022. Available from https://www.unaids.org/en/resources/documents/2022/in-danger-global-aids-update [Accessed: February 12, 2025]

[56] Walker RW, Jusabani A, Aris E, Gray WK, Unwin N, Swai M, et al. Stroke risk factors in an incident population in urban and rural Tanzania: A prospective, community-based, case-control study. The Lancet Global Health. 2013;**1**:e282-e288

[57] GBD 2017 HIV Collaborators. Global, regional, and national incidence, prevalence, and mortality of HIV,

1980-2017, and forecasts to 2030, for 195 countries and territories: A systematic analysis for the global burden of diseases, injuries, and risk factors study 2017. Lancet HIV. 2019;**6**:e831-e859

[58] Sarfo FS, Opare-Sem O, Agyei M, Akassi J, Owusu D, Owolabi M, et al. Risk factors for stroke occurrence in a low HIV endemic West African country: A case-control study. Journal of the Neurological Sciences. 2018;**395**:8-16

[59] Damasceno A, Mayosi BM, Sani M, Ogah OS, Mondo C, Ojji D, et al. The causes, treatment, and outcome of acute heart failure in 1006 Africans from 9 countries. Archives of Internal Medicine. 2012;**172**:1386-1394

[60] Zühlke L, Engel ME, Karthikeyan G, Rangarajan S, Mackie P, Cupido B, et al. Characteristics, complications, and gaps in evidence-based interventions in rheumatic heart disease: The global rheumatic heart disease registry (the REMEDY study). European Heart Journal. 2015;**36**:1115-122a

[61] Fleming HA, Bailey SM. Mitral valve disease, systemic embolism and anticoagulants. Postgraduate Medical Journal. 1971;**47**:599-604

[62] Jauch EC, Saver JL, Adams HP Jr, Bruno A, Connors JJ, Demaerschalk BM, et al. Guidelines for the early management of patients with acute ischemic stroke: A guideline for healthcare professionals from the American Heart Association/ American Stroke Association. Stroke. 2013;**44**:870-947

[63] Deresse B, Shaweno D. Epidemiology and in-hospital outcome of stroke in South Ethiopia. Journal of the Neurological Sciences. 2015;**355**:138-142

[64] Moloi AH, Mall S, Engel ME, Stafford R, Zhu ZW, Zühlke LJ, et al. The health systems barriers and facilitators for RHD prevalence: An epidemiological meta-analysis from Uganda and Tanzania. Global Heart. 2017;**12**:5-15.e3

[65] Wonkam A, Makani J. Sickle cell disease in Africa: An urgent need for longitudinal cohort studies. The Lancet Global Health. 2019;**7**:e1310-e1311

[66] Sarfo FS, Ovbiagele B, Matthew OA, Akpalu A, Wahab K, Obiako R, et al. Antecedent febrile illness and occurrence of stroke in West Africa: The SIREN study. Journal of the Neurological Sciences. 2020;**418**:117158

[67] Cabore JW, Karamagi HC, Kipruto HK, Mungatu JK, Asamani JA, Droti B, et al. COVID-19 in the 47 countries of the WHO African region: A modelling analysis of past trends and future patterns. The Lancet Global Health. 2022;**10**:e1099-e1114

[68] Sarfo FS, Mensah NO, Opoku FA, Adusei-Mensah N, Ampofo M, Ovbiagele B. COVID-19 and stroke: Experience in a Ghanaian healthcare system. Journal of the Neurological Sciences. 2020;**416**:117044

[69] Roushdy T, Hamid E. A review on SARS-CoV-2 and stroke pathogenesis and outcome. Egyptian Journal of Neurology, Psychiatry and Neurosurgery. 2021;**57**:63

[70] The World Bank. Life expectancy at birth—China. Available from: https://data.worldbank.org/indicator/SP.DYN.LE00.IN?locations=CN [Accessed: December 28, 2024]

[71] Ma Q, Li R, Wang L, Yin P, Wang Y, Yan C, et al. Temporal trend and attributable risk factors of stroke burden in China, 1990-2019: An analysis for the global burden of disease study 2019. The Lancet Public Health. 2021;**6**:e897-e906

[72] Tu W-J, Zhao Z, Yin P, Cao L, Zeng J, Chen H, et al. Estimated burden of stroke in China in 2020. JAMA Network Open. 2023;**6**:e231455-e231455

[73] Li Z, Wang C, Zhao X, Liu L, Wang C, Li H, et al. Substantial progress yet significant opportunity for improvement in stroke care in China. Stroke. 2016;**47**:2843-2849

[74] Wu S, Wu B, Liu M, Chen Z, Wang W, Anderson CS, et al. Stroke in China: Advances and challenges in epidemiology, prevention, and management. Lancet Neurology. 2019;**18**:394-405

[75] Luengo-Fernandez R, Paul NL, Gray AM, Pendlebury ST, Bull LM, Welch SJ, et al. Population-based study of disability and institutionalization after transient ischemic attack and stroke: 10-year results of the Oxford vascular study. Stroke. 2013;**44**:2854-2861

[76] Ma J, Tian Z, Chai P, Wan Q, Zhai T, Guo F, et al. Estimating the economic burden of stroke in China: A cost-of-illness study. BMJ Open. 2024;**14**:e080634

[77] Wang W, Jiang B, Sun H, Ru X, Sun D, Wang L, et al. Prevalence, incidence, and mortality of stroke in China: Results from a nationwide population-based survey of 480 687 adults. Circulation. 2017;**135**:759-771

[78] Guan T, Ma J, Li M, Xue T, Lan Z, Guo J, et al. Rapid transitions in the epidemiology of stroke and its risk factors in China from 2002 to 2013. Neurology. 2017;**89**(2017):53-61

[79] Li Y, Yang L, Wang L, Zhang M, Huang Z, Deng Q, et al. Burden of hypertension in China: A nationally representative survey of 174,621 adults. International Journal of Cardiology. 2017;**227**:516-523

[80] Lu Y, Wang P, Zhou T, Lu J, Spatz ES, Nasir K, et al. Comparison of prevalence, awareness, treatment, and control of cardiovascular risk factors in China and the United States. Journal of the American Heart Association. 26 Jan 2018;7(3):e007462

[81] Pan L, Yang Z, Wu Y, Yin RX, Liao Y, Wang J, et al. The prevalence, awareness, treatment and control of dyslipidemia among adults in China. Atherosclerosis. 2016;**248**:2-9

[82] Wang L, Gao P, Zhang M, Huang Z, Zhang D, Deng Q, et al. Prevalence and ethnic pattern of diabetes and prediabetes in China in 2013. JAMA. 2017;**317**:2515-2523

[83] Chen Z, Peto R, Zhou M, Iona A, Smith M, Yang L, et al. Contrasting male and female trends in tobacco-attributed mortality in China: Evidence from successive nationwide prospective cohort studies. Lancet. 2015;**386**:1447-1456

[84] Millwood IY, Li L, Smith M, Guo Y, Yang L, Bian Z, et al. Alcohol consumption in 0.5 million people from 10 diverse regions of China: Prevalence, patterns and socio-demographic and health-related correlates. International Journal of Epidemiology. 2013;**42**:816-827

[85] Tu WJ, Hua Y, Yan F, Bian H, Yang Y, Lou M, et al. Prevalence of stroke in China, 2013-2019: A population-based study. Lancet Regional Health. 2022;**28**:100550

[86] Sun H, Zou X, Liu L. Epidemiological factors of stroke: A survey of the current status in China. Journal of Stroke. 2013;**15**:109-114

[87] Wang Z, Chen Z, Zhang L, Wang X, Hao G, Zhang Z, et al. Status of hypertension in China: Results from the China hypertension survey, 2012-2015. Circulation. 2018;**137**:2344-2356

[88] Li Y, He Y, Lai J, Wang D, Zhang J, Fu P, et al. Dietary patterns are associated with stroke in Chinese adults. The Journal of Nutrition. 2011;**141**:1834-1839

[89] Xue GB, Yu BX, Wang XZ, Wang GQ, Wang ZY. Stroke in urban and rural areas of China. Chinese Medical Journal. 1991;**104**:697-704

[90] Li Y, Jia L, Wu W, Yan J, Liu Y. Urbanization for rural sustainability—Rethinking China's urbanization strategy. Journal of Cleaner Production. 2018;**178**:580-586

[91] Wang M, Luo X, Xu S, Liu W, Ding F, Zhang X, et al. Trends in smoking prevalence and implication for chronic diseases in China: Serial national cross-sectional surveys from 2003 to 2013. The Lancet Respiratory Medicine. 2019;7:35-45

[92] Yu K, Qiu G, Chan KH, Lam KH, Kurmi OP, Bennett DA, et al. Association of solid fuel use with risk of cardiovascular and all-cause mortality in rural China. JAMA. 2018;**319**:1351-1361

[93] Lewicki A. East–west inequalities and the ambiguous racialisation of 'Eastern Europeans'. Journal of Ethnic and Migration Studies. 2023;**49**:1481-1499

[94] Prendes CF, Rantner B, Hamwi T, Stana J, Feigin VL, Stavroulakis K, et al. Burden of stroke in Europe: An analysis of the global burden of disease study findings from 2010 to 2019. Stroke. 2024;**55**:432-442

[95] Dokova KG, Feigin VL. Trends in stroke burden in central and Eastern Europe from 1990-2019. Neuroepidemiology. 2022;**56**:333-344

[96] GBD 2019 Diseases and Injuries Collaborators. Global burden of 369 diseases and injuries in 204 countries and territories, 1990-2019: A systematic analysis for the global burden of disease study 2019. Lancet. 2020;**396**:1204-1222

[97] GBD 2019 Stroke Collaborators. Global, regional, and national burden of stroke and its risk factors, 1990-2019: A systematic analysis for the global burden of disease study 2019. Lancet Neurology. 2021;**20**:795-820

[98] Worldometer. India population. 2024. Available from: https://www.worldometers.info/world-population/india-population/ [Accessed: December 27, 2024]

[99] YA, Sulaja S. Old age mortality in India –an exploration from life expectancy at age 60. International journal of Asian. Social Science. 2016;**6**:698-704

[100] Dalal P, Bhattacharjee M, Vairale J, Bhat P. UN millennium development goals: Can we halt the stroke epidemic in India? Annals of Indian Academy of Neurology. 2007;**10**:130-136

[101] Jones SP, Baqai K, Clegg A, Georgiou R, Harris C, Holland EJ, et al. Stroke in India: A systematic review of the incidence, prevalence, and case fatality. International Journal of Stroke. 2022;**17**:132-140

[102] India State-Level Disease Burden Initiative Neurological Disorders Collaborators. The burden of neurological disorders across the states of India: The global burden of disease study 1990-2019. The Lancet Global Health. 2021;**9**:e1129-e1144

[103] Kamalakannan S, Gudlavalleti ASV, Gudlavalleti VSM, Goenka S, Kuper H. Incidence & prevalence of stroke in India: A systematic review. The

Indian Journal of Medical Research. 2017;**146**:175-185

[104] Tan KS, Pandian JD, Liu L, Toyoda K, Leung TWH, Uchiyama S, et al. Stroke in Asia. Cerebrovascular Diseases Extra. 2024;**14**:58-75

[105] Kapoor M, Agrawal D, Ravi S, Roy A, Subramanian SV, Guleria R. Missing female patients: An observational analysis of sex ratio among outpatients in a referral tertiary care public hospital in India. BMJ Open. 2019;**9**:e026850

[106] Avan A, Digaleh H, Di Napoli M, Stranges S, Behrouz R, Shojaeianbabaei G, et al. Socioeconomic status and stroke incidence, prevalence, mortality, and worldwide burden: An ecological analysis from the global burden of disease study 2017. BMC Medicine. 2019;**17**:191

[107] Singla M, Singh G, Kaur P, Pandian JD. Epidemiology of young stroke in the Ludhiana population-based stroke registry. Annals of Indian Academy of Neurology. 2022;**25**:114-119

[108] Gorthi SP, Garg D. Stroke epidemiology among young persons in India: Every step counts. Annals of Indian Academy of Neurology. 2022;**25**:1-2

[109] Maaijwee NA, Rutten-Jacobs LC, Schaapsmeerders P, van Dijk EJ, de Leeuw FE. Ischaemic stroke in young adults: Risk factors and long-term consequences. Nature Reviews. Neurology. 2014;**10**:315-325

[110] Ke C, Gupta R, Xavier D, Prabhakaran D, Mathur P, Kalkonde YV, et al. Divergent trends in ischaemic heart disease and stroke mortality in India from 2000 to 2015: A nationally representative mortality study. The Lancet Global Health. 2018;**6**(2018):e914-e923

[111] Holmstedt CA, Turan TN, Chimowitz MI. Atherosclerotic intracranial arterial stenosis: Risk factors, diagnosis, and treatment. Lancet Neurology. 2013;**12**:1106-1114

[112] Pandian JD, Padma Srivastava MV, Aaron S, Ranawaka UK, Venketasubramanian N, Sebastian IA, et al. The burden, risk factors and unique etiologies of stroke in South-East Asia region (SEAR). Lancet Regional Health Southeast Asia. 2023;**17**:100290

[113] Wang S, Zou XL, Wu LX, Zhou HF, Xiao L, Yao T, et al. Epidemiology of intracerebral hemorrhage: A systematic review and meta-analysis. Frontiers in Neurology. 2022;**13**:915813

[114] Aaron S, Lakshmanan J, Sudarsanam TD, Benjamin K, Durairaj J, Mathew V, et al. Cerebral venous thrombosis, seasonal trends, and climatic influence: A region-specificstudy. Annals of Indian Academy of Neurology. 2020;**23**:522-527

[115] Wasay M, Kaul S, Menon B, Dai AI, Saadatnia M, Malik A, et al. Asian study of cerebral venous thrombosis. Journal of Stroke and Cerebrovascular Diseases. 2019;**28**:104247

[116] Aaron S, Alexander M, Maya T, Mathew V, Goel M, Nair SC, et al. Underlying prothrombotic states in pregnancy associated cerebral venous thrombosis. Neurology India. 2010;**58**:555-559

[117] D. World Health Organization. Noncommunicable, and C. Mental Health. WHO STEPS Stroke Manual: The WHO STEPwise Approach to

Stroke Surveillance / Noncommunicable Diseases and Mental Health. Geneva: World Health Organization, World Health Organization; 2005

[118] Worldometer. South America and the Caribbean population 2024. Available from https://www.worldometers.info/world-population/latin-america-and-the-caribbean-population/ [Accessed: January 24, 2025]

[119] Muñoz-Venturelli P, González F, Urrutia F, Mazzon E, Navia V, Brunser A, et al. Stroke care and collaborative academic research in Latin America. Salud Pública de México. 2022;**64**:S40-s45

[120] Cagna-Castillo D, Salcedo-Carrillo AL, Carrillo-Larco RM, Bernabé-Ortiz A. Prevalence and incidence of stroke in Latin America and the Caribbean: A systematic review and meta-analysis. Scientific Reports. 2023;**13**:6809

[121] Delfino C, Nuñez M, Asenjo-Lobos C, Gonzalez F, Riviotta A, Urrutia F, et al. Stroke in Latin America: Systematic review of incidence, prevalence, and case-fatality in 1997-2021. International Journal of Stroke. 2023;**18**:645-656

[122] Saposnik G, Del Brutto OH. Stroke in South America: A systematic review of incidence, prevalence, and stroke subtypes. Stroke. 2003;**34**:2103-2107

[123] Pacheco-Barrios K, Giannoni-Luza S, Navarro-Flores A, Rebello-Sanchez I, Parente J, Balbuena A, et al. Burden of stroke and population-attributable fractions of risk factors in Latin America and the Caribbean. Journal of the American Heart Association. 2022;**11**:e027044

[124] Nuñez M, Delfino C, Asenjo-Lobos C, Schilling A, Lavados P, Anderson CS, et al. Disparities in stroke incidence over time by sex and age in Latin America and the Caribbean region 1997 to 2021: A systematic review and meta-analysis. Journal of the American Heart Association. 2023;**12**:e029800

[125] Gonzalez-Aquines A, Rosales J, De Souza AC, Corredor-Quintero A, Barboza MA, Navia-Gonzalez V, et al. Availability and barriers to access post-stroke rehabilitation in Latin America. Journal of Stroke and Cerebrovascular Diseases. 2024;**33**:107917

[126] Dittrich LB, da Silva Etges APB, de Souza JS, Marcolino MAZ, Rocha E, Amaya P, et al. Cost evaluation of acute ischemic stroke in Latin America: A multicentric study. Lancet Regional Health. 2025;**41**:100959

[127] W. Bank. East Asia and Pacific Economic Update, October 2022: Reforms for Recovery. Washington, DC, United States: The World Bank Group; 2022

[128] Feigin VL, Johnson CO, Roth GA, Bisignano C, Abady GG, Abbasifard M, et al. Global, regional, and national burden of stroke and its risk factors, 1990-2019: A systematic analysis for the global burden of disease study 2019. Lancet Neurology. 2021;**20**:795-820

[129] W.H. Organization. Global Status Report on Noncommunicable Diseases 2021. Geneva: World Health Organization; 2021

[130] Harris S, Sungkar S, Rasyid A, Kurniawan M, Mesiano T, Hidayat R. TOAST subtypes of ischemic stroke and its risk factors: A hospital-based study at Cipto Mangunkusumo hospital, Indonesia. Stroke Research and Treatment. 2018;**2018**:9589831

[131] Sharma VK, Tsivgoulis G, Teoh HL, Ong BK, Chan BP. Stroke risk factors and outcomes among various Asian

ethnic groups in Singapore. Journal of Stroke and Cerebrovascular Diseases. 2012;**21**:299-304

[132] Rattanawong W, Hemachudha P, Anukoolwittaya P, Pongpitakmetha T. Cerebral Gnathostomiasis: An unusual course of recurrent hemorrhagic stroke. Annals of Neurology. 2022;**92**:107-109

[133] Li HM, Huang YK, Su YC, Kao CH. Risk of stroke in patients with dengue fever: A population-based cohort study. CMAJ. 2018;**190**:E285-e290

[134] Koge J, Shiozawa M, Toyoda K. Acute stroke care in the With-COVID-19 era: Experience at a comprehensive stroke center in Japan. Frontiers in Neurology. 2020;**11**:611504

[135] Tang LL, Chen WQ, Xue WQ, He YQ, Zheng RS, Zeng YX, et al. Global trends in incidence and mortality of nasopharyngeal carcinoma. Cancer Letters. 2016;**374**:22-30

[136] Lee GH, Lim MP, DeSilva WEH, Chang HM. Long term outcome of patients with symptomatic severe carotid stenosis who receive carotid artery angioplasty and stenting: A comparison between prior and no irradiation. International Journal of Stroke. 2014;**9**:137

[137] Liao W, Zheng Y, Bi S, Zhang B, Xiong Y, Li Y, et al. Carotid stenosis prevalence after radiotherapy in nasopharyngeal carcinoma: A meta-analysis. Radiotherapy and Oncology. 2019;**133**:167-175

[138] Singhania N, Bansal S, Nimmatoori DP, Ejaz AA, McCullough PA, Singhania G. Current overview on hypercoagulability in COVID-19. American Journal of Cardiovascular Drugs. 2020;**20**:393-403

[139] Tang X, Zheng F. A review of ischemic stroke in COVID-19: Currently known pathophysiological mechanisms. Neurological Sciences. 2022;**43**:67-79

[140] Spence JD, de Freitas GR, Pettigrew LC, Ay H, Liebeskind DS, Kase CS, et al. Mechanisms of stroke in COVID-19. Cerebrovascular Diseases. 2020;**49**:451-458

[141] Pandian JD, Panagos PD, Sebastian IA, Silva GS, Furie KL, Liu L, et al. Maintaining stroke care during the COVID-19 pandemic in lower- and middle-income countries: World stroke organization position statement endorsed by American Stroke Association and American Heart Association. Stroke. 2022;**53**:1043-1050

Chapter 3

Socio-Economic Inequalities in Stroke: A Global Perspective

Olaleye Akinmola Adeniji and Ayotomiwa Fagbemi

Abstract

The effects of socio-economic inequalities on stroke risk, clinical profile, and outcomes continue to attract global public health interest. This is because, despite impressive advances in stroke prevention and acute care, substantial heterogeneities remain with regard to stroke incidence, prevalence, prevention, treatment and outcomes across many parts of the world. Socio-economic factors may influence differences in access to resources, lifestyle and behavioral choices, psychosocial stressors and the built environment and may partly explain why these heterogeneities persist. The political and cultural environment in which people live, grow and work is also critical in shaping policy priorities and subsequent allocation of resources to non-communicable diseases such as stroke. In this chapter, an overview of the effects of socio-economic inequalities on stroke risk factors, incidence, prevalence, mortality, is provided. Potential strategies for advancing equity in stroke care, especially across diverse populations, are also discussed.

Keywords: socio-economic inequalities, stroke, low socio-economic status, disparities, social determinants

1. Introduction

Stroke is a major disabling disease of global public health importance. It is the second leading cause of death and third leading cause of adult-onset disability globally [1]. Stroke outcomes such as death, disability, dementia, depression and anxiety are major contributors to increased costs of care, caregiver burden and poor quality of life among stroke survivors and their families [2, 3]. Over the years, understanding of stroke risk factors, clinical presentation, outcomes and global burden has increased in tandem with impressive advances in stroke prevention, care and treatment. However, despite these, substantial heterogeneity exists in the global stroke burden [1]. This may be partly because of socio-economic factors prevalent within the population and among individuals that influence stroke epidemiology and outcomes [4]. These factors sometimes also called social determinants of health (SDOH), have become of increasing interest in global public health [4]. The World Health Organization (WHO) Commission on the SDOH in 2010 defined SDOH as non-medical factors that influence health outcomes [5]. These include *structural* factors such as the political, legal, economic, educational and cultural policies or beliefs prevalent within societies that determine the gradients of income, education, occupation or social class [6]. These structural factors play an important role in shaping the material, biological and psychosocial living situation of the individual or society including factors such as housing, food availability, early childhood factors, the lived environment, physical activity and mental well-being. These "downstream" factors are referred to as *intermediate* determinants of health [6]. The accretionary effects of these structural and intermediary determinants play a critical role in shaping differences in stroke risk within populations (inequalities) and eventual outcomes after stroke (disparities) [7] (**Figure 1**) . A better understanding of the drivers of these determinants has, however, emerged, highlighting a strong association between low socio-economic status (a composite metric including many indices such as level of education, neighborhood socio-economic status and income level) and stroke risk and outcomes [8–10] and are reviewed in this chapter. Based on these, some strategies for addressing these inequalities in population stroke prevention and care have been suggested and are also reviewed.

1.1 Stroke risk factors

Low socio-economic status (SES) is an important driver of inequalities in stroke risk from many studies [11–14]. The overall effects of modifiable stroke risk factors such as hypertension, diabetes mellitus, obesity, sedentary lifestyle, and alcohol and tobacco use have a strong correlation with low SES in both high-income countries (HICs) [11] and low- and middle-income countries (LMICs) [4]. The association between low SES and dyslipidemia has also been reported [15]. High SES has also been documented as a risk factor for stroke [16], although overall low SES seems to be associated with more severe strokes than high SES [4]. This may be because higher SES increases the adoption of urbanization, lifestyles and diets that increase the risk of stroke.

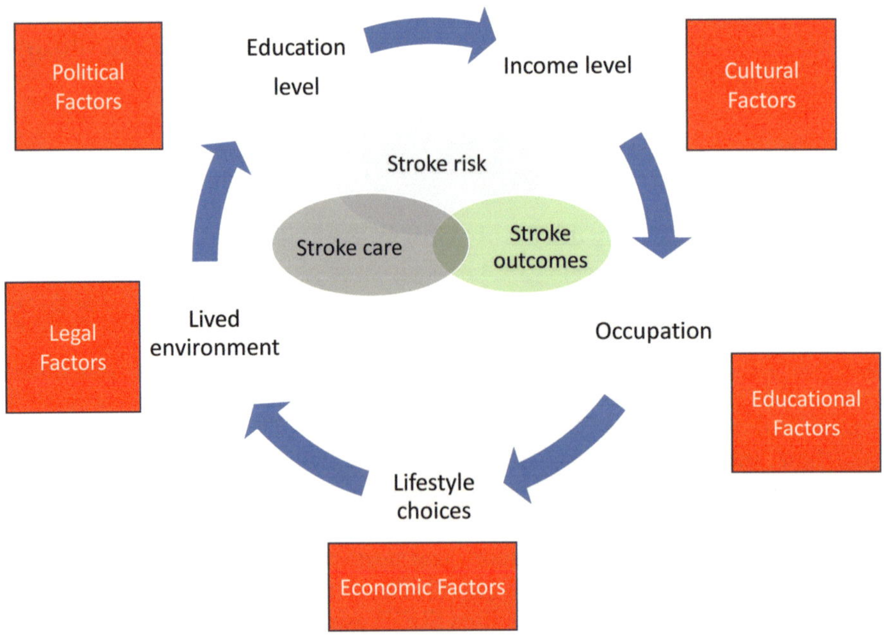

Figure 1.
A diagram showing the interaction between structural (red squares) and intermediate determinants of health (text) and stroke risk, stroke care and outcomes (Venn diagram).

Although the definitions of low SES vary across different studies [11], a consistent pattern of higher stroke risk with increasing indices of low SES has been reported [11, 13, 14]. Several other indices of low SES such as unemployment status [12], rural habitation [17], non-serviced accommodation [17], low educational level [18] and lack of health insurance [19] have also been associated with higher risks of stroke. These associations seem to be present within both HICs and LMICs [11, 18, 19], suggesting that stroke risk factors may be driven by similar socio-economic variables across diverse populations. Data from the Global Burden of Disease Investigators (2019) also suggest that low SES is strongly associated with the risk of stroke and stroke burden [1].

The effects of SES on stroke risk may even be more pronounced in certain ethnic groups. In the United States, for example, people of African Ancestry have a higher incidence of stroke, more severe strokes and higher stroke mortality than other racial groups and this risk has persisted despite an overall reduction in stroke incidence in the general population over the last five decades [20, 21]. Markers of low SES such as low income have been reported as associated with a higher risk of stroke among African Americans compared to other ethnic groups although other factors such as genetic and epigenetic factors have also been suggested [21]. In the REGARDS trial, for example, each additional SDOH factor was associated with higher odds of stroke, especially in individuals under 75 years of age [22].

The pathways by which low SES increases stroke risk factors such as hypertension, diabetes, obesity, poor nutrition, sedentary lifestyle, alcohol and tobacco consumption among low SES populations are likely complex and multifaceted. Stroke knowledge and awareness has been reported to be poorer among people with low SES [23], and this may lead to poor health-seeking behavior. The burden of infectious diseases such as HIV has also been reported to be higher among people with low SES, and this may impact stroke risk, especially in regions of high HIV endemicity [24]. Further, structural and intermediate barriers to equitable access to health appear more prevalent among people with low SES. People with low SES, especially in LMICs, have higher out-of-pocket expenditures and higher rates of catastrophic health expenditure (a marker of impoverization due to illness) due to stroke [25]. These barriers may prevent early presentation and treatment of stroke risk factors and poorer outcomes.

1.2 Early life factors

Markers of low SES in early life, such as inadequate nutrition, lower parental social class and poor social mobility, have also been associated with increased stroke risk [26]. These markers may influence stroke risk across the life course. The fetal origins hypothesis by Barker [27], which highlights how adverse early life factors such as poor nutrition increase the risk of cardiovascular diseases such as stroke in later life, is relevant in linking adverse early life factors to increased stroke risk in later life. Studies suggest that individuals with anthropomorphic indices of inadequate nutrition such as low birth weight, pre-term birth and short stature have an increased risk of stroke risk factors such as hypertension, diabetes and obesity in later life [26, 28]. Paternal social class and a positive family history of stroke death have also been associated with increased stroke risk [29, 30]. Inter-generational social mobility has also been associated with increased risk of ischemic stroke with downward social mobility especially between adolescence and early adulthood being associated with higher odds of stroke in later life [31].

1.3 Stroke incidence

According to the GBD investigators 2021 [1], stroke incidence seems to be increasing globally. Stroke incidence increased, especially in parts of Southeast Asia and Oceania [1], from 1990 to 2020. This contrasted with the picture in 2017, when there was an overall 11.3% decline in age-standardized stroke incidence globally [4]. This observed increase in stroke incidence was seen mostly in young to middle-aged people. Notably, from the 2021 study, there was a strong association between increasing stroke incidence and lower socio-demographic indices (SDIs) [1]. The major drivers of increasing stroke incidence include demographic factors such as increasing aging of the population, stroke risk factors such as uncontrolled hypertension, poor lifestyle choices (obesity, smoking, alcohol use and sedentary lifestyle) and air pollution [1]. These factors act in synergy with other system factors such as absence or poorly developed stroke prevention and treatment services, inadequate stroke care manpower and low levels of public spending on healthcare.

Generally, stroke incidence appears to be higher among people with markers of low SES such as low level of education, low-income status and low neighborhood social class [11, 14]. This is likely due to the higher burden of stroke risk factors and poor screening and treatment among people with low SES.

1.4 Stroke prevalence

Age-standardized stroke prevalence seems to have doubled over the past 30 years despite advances in prevention and treatment of stroke [1, 4]. This trend of increasing stroke prevalence seems to be predominant in LMICs [4]. The relationship between low SES and stroke prevalence in LMICs also seems to be non-linear, however, with increasing stroke prevalence at both high and lower ends of the socio-economic strata [32, 33]. People with low SES in urban areas appear to have a higher prevalence of stroke compared to those in rural areas [33].

1.5 Stroke mortality

It is estimated that global stroke mortality will increase by 50% from 2020 to 2050, and a substantial part of this mortality burden would be borne by LMICs [34]. Already, LMICs bear a disproportionate burden of stroke mortality while having the least number of human resources to tackle it [1, 34]. According to the Global Burden of Diseases Injuries and Risk Investigators 2021 [1], 87.2% of all fatal strokes, and 89.4% of all stroke-related Disability-Adjusted Life-Years (DALYs) occurred in all low-income and middle-income countries (LMICs) combined in 2021. The drivers of increasing stroke mortality include absent or poorly developed acute stroke treatment services, poorly developed pre-hospital stroke services and huge financial barriers to accessing acute stroke care due to absence of universal health coverage [34]. Although data on specific racial, gender and socio-economic disparities in stroke mortality in LMICs is still emerging, their overall effects are likely to be significant due to challenges with resources available for healthcare and non-communicable disease prevention. In contrast, HICs have experienced a progressive decline in stroke mortality [35, 36]. This decline in stroke mortality in HICs occurred despite increasing aging in many of these countries [37, 38]. The main drivers of reducing stroke mortality in HICs likely include relatively reduced stroke incidence (due to systematic improvements in population health and population stroke risk factor control) and reduced stroke case-fatality rates (due to advances in acute stroke treatments such as thrombolysis and mechanical thrombectomy for ischemic strokes, decompression and evacuation surgeries for hemorrhagic strokes and the uptake of acute stroke units) [35–38]. In many HICs, these declines in stroke mortality have been accompanied by concomitant declines in mortality from ischemic heart disease and dementia, suggesting a pragmatic model for the control of not just stroke but other NCDs as well [39].

2. Equity-based approaches to reducing socio-economic inequalities

Health equity is defined as the reduction or elimination of all remediable or unfair differences in health and health outcomes among different social, ethnic, gender, religious and geographic population groups [40] and has become a topical issue in public health. The concept is relevant to stroke prevention and care because of the effect of socio-economic inequalities on stroke risk and outcomes. Despite the advances in stroke prevention and acute stroke care over the past decades, the promise of access to safe, timely, effective, affordable and high-quality stroke care remains challenging for diverse populations due to systemic and structural barriers from differences in race or ethnicity, gender, economic class or educational level. A range of solutions has been proposed and operationalized within different models of stroke care with a view to reducing some of the observed disparities in stroke. Many of these solutions have their strengths and weaknesses, but they provide useful templates for advancing equity in stroke care and are discussed below.

2.1 Stroke surveillance and prevention

Stroke surveillance refers to systematic attempts by communities or countries to map the risk factors for stroke within populations including regular surveys of populations at risk with a view to early screening and treatment of these stroke risk factors [41]. It is an important component of the stroke quadrangle [41] (comprising stroke surveillance, prevention, acute treatment and rehabilitation). These attempts may involve mass surveys of populations at risk with a focus on identifying stroke risk factors and determining individual risks. Stroke prevention also involves strategies to modify the population determinants of stroke risk factors and to prevent the establishment of these risk factors (primordial prevention) or strategies to actively treat those populations who already have stroke risk factors to prevent the occurrence of a stroke (primary prevention) [42]. These (primordial and primary prevention) may involve public legislation and educational programs, bans and taxes on tobacco and alcohol products, physical activity campaigns and active screening and treatment of stroke risk factors by trained staff usually at the primary level of care (population-based strategy) [42]. A second strategy involves identification of individuals or population subgroups particularly at high risk of stroke (high-risk strategy) [43]. While population-based approaches are thought to be more cost effective, questions remain about feasibility and sustainability [43]. High-risk strategy of screening and treatment relies mostly on individual risk-stratification and treatment of high-risk individuals [43].

Digital tools for stroke risk stratification have also been developed and used [44]. One of the more commonly known and widely recommended tools is the Stroke Risko-meter Application [45]. However, many of the currently available risk-stratification models, including the Stroke Risko-meter Application, do not include markers of Socio-economic status or SDOH. Further, these applications were derived from specific populations and may therefore underestimate or overestimate stroke risk in non-derived populations [44, 45]. Tele-health tools such as the Stroke Coach have also been studied as a pragmatic means of screening and identifying at-risk populations, disseminating stroke knowledge and promoting healthy lifestyle and behavioral choices such as smoking cessation and tobacco use cessation [46]. There is evidence that these tele-health tools may be effective at improving glycemic control, dyslipidemia and weight loss [47]. However, their overall efficacy in reducing stroke risk is still being investigated.

Challenges facing digital approaches to stroke primary prevention include the digital health divide between HICs and LMICs, structural barriers such as availability of telephony infrastructure in rural areas, broadband challenges and costs [44, 45]. Many of these digital tools require some level of literacy or numeracy which may also be a challenge in low-literacy populations.

2.1.1 Task shifting and sharing

Task shifting is defined as the systematic transfer of primary care duties from physicians to non-physician healthcare workers, such as nurses, pharmacists or community health workers [48]. Task shifting may be a pragmatic approach where there are no physicians. However, in areas with low physician densities, task sharing involving appropriately trained and certified non-physician health workers may be useful in assisting the physician to deliver healthcare services [48]. Task-sharing strategies have been reported to be feasible and effective in improving the screening and management of stroke risk factors in community settings [49]. Data from many studies and meta-analyses suggest that task sharing with non-physician health workers is effective for the management of blood pressure and diabetes mellitus in both community and hospital-based settings in both HICs and LMICs [50–52]. However, many gaps remain in effectively deploying this strategy at scale [51]. The effectiveness of a task-sharing strategy in improving overall cardiovascular risks is also under investigation.

3. Future directions and conclusion

As research on the socio-economic inequalities in stroke care and outcomes continues to grow, priorities for improving these inequalities will become of increasing political and economic interest, in tandem with the projected increase in global stroke burden. Therefore, accurate characterization of the impact of different socio-economic determinants of health within diverse populations will be key for research, clinical practice and policy implementation. Delineating the effect sizes of various SDOH using highly rigorous methods will also be important to provide insights into the best areas to concentrate public health resources. Implementation strategies to improve these SDOH will also be critical. Endpoints such as feasibility, sustainability and cost-effectiveness of these interventions will be important indices. Overall, political will and multi-sectoral strategies will be important determinants of respective countries outcomes in the efforts to improve these markers of socio-economic inequalities and optimize stroke care and outcomes for vulnerable populations.

DOI: http://dx.doi.org/10.5772/intechopen.1010685

Author details

Olaleye Akinmola Adeniji[1*] and Ayotomiwa Fagbemi[2]

1 Department of Neurology, University College Hospital, Ibadan, Oyo State, Nigeria

2 Neurology Unit, Federal Medical Center, Abeokuta, Ogun State, Nigeria

*Address all correspondence to: leyeadeniji@yahoo.co.uk

References

[1] Feigin VL, Abate MD, Abate YH, Abd ElHafeez S, Abd-Allah F, Abdelalim A, et al. Global, regional, and national burden of stroke and its risk factors, 1990-2021: A systematic analysis for the Global Burden of Disease Study 2021. The Lancet Neurology. 2024;**23**(10):973-1003

[2] Gorelick PB. The global burden of stroke: Persistent and disabling. The Lancet Neurology. 2019;**18**(5):417-418

[3] Lanas F, Seron P. Facing the stroke burden worldwide. The Lancet Global Health. 2021;**9**(3):e235-e236

[4] Avan A, Digaleh H, Di Napoli M, Stranges S, Behrouz R, Shojaeianbabaei G, et al. Socioeconomic status and stroke incidence, prevalence, mortality, and worldwide burden: An ecological analysis from the Global Burden of Disease Study 2017. BMC Medicine. 2019;**17**(1):1-30

[5] Solar O, Irwin A. A conceptual framework for action on the social determinants of health. (Social determinants of health discussion paper 2 (policy and practice)). Geneva, Switzerland: WHO; 2010. [September 22, 2016]. Available from: http://www.who.int/sdhconference/resources/ConceptualframeworkforactiononSDH_eng.pdf [Accessed: 19th May 2025]

[6] Williams GH. The determinants of health: Structure, context and agency. Sociology of Health & Illness. 2003;**25**(3):131-154

[7] Ovbiagele B. Decoding stroke disparities: Zip codes, color codes, and epigenetic codes. Transactions of the American Clinical and Climatological Association. 2024;**134**:214

[8] Pantoja-Ruiz C, Akinyemi R, Lucumi-Cuesta DI, Youkee D, Emmett E, Soley-Bori M, et al. Socioeconomic status and stroke: A review of the latest evidence on inequalities and their drivers. Stroke. 2025;**56**:794-805

[9] Sommer I, Griebler U, Mahlknecht P, Thaler K, Bouskill K, Gartlehner G, et al. Socioeconomic inequalities in non-communicable diseases and their risk factors: An overview of systematic reviews. BMC Public Health. 2015;**15**:1-2

[10] Cox AM, McKevitt C, Rudd AG, Wolfe CD. Socioeconomic status and stroke. The Lancet Neurology. 2006;**5**(2):181-188

[11] Marshall IJ, Wang Y, Crichton S, McKevitt C, Rudd AG, Wolfe CD. The effects of socioeconomic status on stroke risk and outcomes. The Lancet Neurology. 2015;**14**(12):1206-1218

[12] Avendano M, Kawachi I, Van Lenthe F, Boshuizen HC, Mackenbach JP, Van den Bos GA, et al. Socioeconomic status and stroke incidence in the US elderly: The role of risk factors in the EPESE study. Stroke. 2006;**37**(6):1368-1373

[13] Kumar A, Prasad M, Kathuria P, Nair P, Pandit AK, Sahu JK, et al. Low socioeconomic status is an independent risk factor for ischemic stroke: A case-control study in North Indian population. Neuroepidemiology. 2015;**44**(3):138-143

[14] Amarenco P, Abboud H, Labreuche J, Arauz A, Bryer A, Lavados PM, et al. Impact of living and socioeconomic characteristics on cardiovascular risk in ischemic stroke patients. International Journal of Stroke. 2014;**9**(8):1065-1072

[15] Pirillo A, Casula M, Olmastroni E, Norata GD, Catapano AL. Global epidemiology of dyslipidaemias. Nature Reviews Cardiology. 2021;**18**(10):689-700

[16] Yamanie N, Sjaaf AC, Felistia Y, Susanto NH, Diana A, Lamuri A, et al. High socioeconomic status is associated with stroke severity among stroke patients in the National Brain Centre Hospital, Jakarta, Indonesia. Preventive Medicine Reports. 2023;**32**:102170

[17] Singh GK, Siahpush M, Azuine RE, Williams SD. Increasing area deprivation and socioeconomic inequalities in heart disease, stroke, and cardiovascular disease mortality among working age populations, United States, 1969-2011. International Journal of MCH and AIDS. 2015;**3**(2):119

[18] McHutchison CA, Backhouse EV, Cvoro V, Shenkin SD, Wardlaw JM. Education, socioeconomic status, and intelligence in childhood and stroke risk in later life: A meta-analysis. Epidemiology. 2017;**28**(4):608-618

[19] Shen JJ, Washington EL. Disparities in outcomes among patients with stroke associated with insurance status. Stroke. 2007;**38**(3):1010-1016

[20] Addo J, Ayerbe L, Mohan KM, Crichton S, Sheldenkar A, Chen R, et al. Socioeconomic status and stroke: An updated review. Stroke. 2012;**43**(4): 1186-1191

[21] Towfighi A, Ovbiagele B. Health equity and actionable disparities in stroke: Understanding and problem-solving 2023 update. Journal of the American Heart Association. 2024;**13**(7):e031306

[22] Reshetnyak E, Ntamatungiro M, Pinheiro LC, Howard VJ, Carson AP, Martin KD, et al. Impact of multiple social determinants of health on incident stroke. Stroke. 2020;**51**(8):2445-2453

[23] Jones SP, Jenkinson AJ, Leathley MJ, Watkins CL. Stroke knowledge and awareness: An integrative review of the evidence. Age and Ageing. 2010;**39**(1):11-22

[24] Wojcicki JM. Socioeconomic status as a risk factor for HIV infection in women in East, Central and Southern Africa: A systematic review. Journal of Biosocial Science. 2005;**37**(1):1-36

[25] Rochmah TN, Rahmawati IT, Dahlui M, Budiarto W, Bilqis N. Economic burden of stroke disease: A systematic review. International Journal of Environmental Research and Public Health. 2021;**18**(14):7552

[26] Lilja L, Bygdell M, Martikainen J, Rosengren A, Ohlsson C, Kindblom JM. Low birth weight as an early-life risk factor for adult stroke among men. The Journal of Pediatrics. 2021;**237**:162-167

[27] Barker DJ, Godfrey KM, Gluckman PD, Harding JE, Owens JA, Robinson JS. Fetal nutrition and cardiovascular disease in adult life. The Lancet. 1993;**341**(8850):938-941

[28] Tabara Y, Shoji-Asahina A, Ogawa A, Sato Y. Additive association of blood pressure and short stature with stroke incidence in 450,000 Japanese adults: The Shizuoka study. Hypertension Research. 2024;**47**:2075-2085

[29] Wannamethee SG, Whincup PH, Shaper G, Walker M. Influence of fathers' social class on cardiovascular disease in middle-aged men. The Lancet. 1996;**348**(9037):1259-1263

[30] Wannamethee SG, Shaper AG, Ebrahim S. History of parental death

from stroke or heart trouble and the risk of stroke in middle-aged men. Stroke. 1996;**27**(9):1492-1498

[31] Grau AJ, Aigner A, Urbanek C, Palm F, Buggle F, Safer A, et al. Socioeconomic decline and advancement within and between generations and the risk of stroke-a case-control study. Neurological Research and Practice. 2019;**1**:1-6

[32] Ekenze OS, Birinus Adikaibe EA, Obinna O, Peter C, Casmir O, Nkiruka OP, et al. The prevalence of stroke survivors in urban slums in Enugu, Nigeria. Open Journal of Preventive Medicine. 2019;**9**(06):51-67

[33] Engels T, Baglione Q, Audibert M, Viallefont A, Mourji F, El Alaoui Faris M, et al. Socioeconomic status and stroke prevalence in Morocco: Results from the Rabat-Casablanca study. PLoS ONE. 2014;**9**(2):e89271

[34] Feigin VL, Owolabi MO, Abd-Allah F, Akinyemi RO, Bhattacharjee NV, Brainin M, et al. Pragmatic solutions to reduce the global burden of stroke: A World Stroke Organization–Lancet Neurology Commission. The Lancet Neurology. 2023;**22**(12):1160-1206

[35] Soto Á, Guillén-Grima F, Morales G, Muñoz S, Aguinaga-Ontoso I. Trends in mortality from stroke in the European Union, 1996-2015. European Journal of Neurology. 2021;**28**(1):182-191

[36] Wafa HA, Wolfe CD, Emmett E, Roth GA, Johnson CO, Wang Y. Burden of stroke in Europe: Thirty-year projections of incidence, prevalence, deaths, and disability-adjusted life years. Stroke. 2020;**51**(8):2418-2427

[37] Rand K, Dahl FA, Viana J, Rønning OM, Faiz KW, Barra M. Fewer ischemic strokes, despite an ageing population: Stroke models from observed incidence in Norway 2010-2015. BMC Health Services Research. 2019;**19**:1-1

[38] Ananth CV, Brandt JS, Keyes KM, Graham HL, Kostis JB, Kostis WJ. Epidemiology and trends in stroke mortality in the USA, 1975-2019. International Journal of Epidemiology. 2023;**52**(3):858-866

[39] Avan A, Aamodt AH, Selbæk G, Bovim G, Bassetti CL, Boon P, et al. Decreasing incidence of stroke, ischaemic heart disease and dementia in Norway, 1990-2019, a Global Burden of Disease study: An opportunity. European Journal of Neurology. 2023;**30**(8):2267-2277

[40] Braveman P. Health disparities and health equity: Concepts and measurement. Annual Review of Public Health. 2006;**27**(1):167-194

[41] Owolabi MO. Taming the burgeoning stroke epidemic in Africa: Stroke quadrangle to the rescue. The West Indian Medical Journal. 2011;**60**(4):412-421

[42] Adeniji O, Olowoyo P, Akinyemi R, Fisher M, Owolabi M. Advances in primordial, primary, and secondary prevention of stroke in diverse populations. Stroke. 2024;**55**:2359-2365

[43] Owolabi MO, Thrift AG, Mahal A, Ishida M, Martins S, Johnson WD, et al. Primary stroke prevention worldwide: Translating evidence into action. The Lancet Public Health. 2022;**7**(1):e74-e85

[44] Feigin VL, Owolabi M, Hankey GJ, Pandian J, Martins SC. Digital health in primordial and primary stroke prevention: A systematic review. Stroke. 2022;**53**(3):1008-1019

[45] Parmar P, Krishnamurthi R, Ikram MA, Hofman A, Mirza SS, Varakin Y, et al. The Stroke Riskometer™ app: Validation of a data collection tool and stroke risk predictor. International Journal of Stroke. 2015;**10**(2):231-244

[46] Sakakibara BM, Lear SA, Barr SI, Goldsmith CH, Schneeberg A, Silverberg ND, et al. Telehealth coaching to improve self-management for secondary prevention after stroke: A randomized controlled trial of Stroke Coach. International Journal of Stroke. 2022;**17**(4):455-464

[47] Merriel SW, Andrews V, Salisbury C. Telehealth interventions for primary prevention of cardiovascular disease: A systematic review and meta-analysis. Preventive Medicine. 2014;**64**:88-95

[48] World Health Organization (WHO). Task shifting: rational redistribution of task among health workforce teams: global recommendations and guidelines. Geneva, Switzerland: WHO; 2008. Available from: https://iris.who.int/bitstream/handle/10665/43821/9789241596312_eng.pdf [Accessed: 19th May 2025]

[49] Maria JL, Anand TN, Dona B, Prinu J, Prabhakaran D, Jeemon P. Task-sharing interventions for improving control of diabetes in low-income and middle-income countries: A systematic review and meta-analysis. The Lancet Global Health. 2021;**9**(2):e170-e180

[50] Mirhoseiny S, Geelvink T, Martin S, Vollmar HC, Stock S, Redaelli M. Does task delegation to non-physician health professionals improve quality of diabetes care? Results of a scoping review. PLoS ONE. 2019;**14**(10):e0223159

[51] Van der Wees PJ, Friedberg MW, Guzman EA, Ayanian JZ, Rodriguez HP. Comparing the implementation of team approaches for improving diabetes care in community health centers. BMC Health Services Research. 2014;**14**:1

[52] Pandian JD, Kalkonde Y, Sebastian IA, Felix C, Urimubenshi G, Bosch J. Stroke systems of care in low-income and middle-income countries: Challenges and opportunities. The Lancet. 2020;**396**(10260):1443-1451

Chapter 4

Young Stroke: Epidemiology and Etiology

Neetika Sharma and Ashish Sharma

Abstract

Stroke is the second leading cause of death in the world. Young stroke is considered at an age of less than 45 years. The incidence of young stroke ranges from 7 to 15 in 100,000 people per year. This incidence has substantially increased and adds to the cost of long-term care, posing a huge challenge to the health care system. As with stroke in normal adults, causes of stroke in the young also include large artery atherosclerosis, cardioembolic, small vessel disease, other determined etiology, and undetermined etiology. Identification of rare causes of young stroke requires a major diagnostic effort. Which diagnostic test is necessary for each patient is a matter that needs to be decided individually. Among the other determined and undetermined etiologies, non-atherosclerotic vasculopathy and genetic stroke syndromes constitute the major causes of stroke. Young females are more predisposed to migraine with aura, vascular disorders, and autoimmune conditions. Ethnic disparity also exists in this subset of the population. Lifestyle choices (cigarette smoking, drug abuse, and a sedentary lifestyle) can significantly increase the rate of stroke among the young. Causes of stroke in the young are often missed. With advances in science, it has become easier to detect genetic causes of stroke, as they have different management and their prognosis varies.

Keywords: young stroke, genetic stroke syndrome, juvenile stroke, global stroke burden, causes of young stroke

1. Introduction

Traditionally, stroke is considered a disease of the elderly; however, stroke at a young age < 50 years makes up to 10% of all strokes and is still rising [1]. With the global rise in incidences of metabolic disorders like diabetes, hypertension, dyslipidemia, obesity with smoking, drug abuse, physical inactivity, and heart diseases, the prevalence of young stroke has increased. Young adults of all races and ethnicities are affected [2]. Stroke adds to morbidity and affects the quality of life. Apart from neurological conditions, patients also have to deal with psychosocial consequences. In this chapter, we will discuss the epidemiology along with common and uncommon but important causes of stroke in the young population.

1.1 Epidemiology

The incidence of ischemic stroke among young adults is rising globally. A 27-year-long study from France found that the incidence of stroke for those <55 years of age was 20.2 per 100,000 adults in 2003–2011 [3]. In the United States, the incidence of stroke for the age group 20–44 was 28 per 100,000 in 2015 [4]. The incidence of young stroke varies from continent to continent. In Europe, it ranges from 7 to 8 per 100,000 to 100 per 100,000 in Sub-Saharan Africa [5]. Slight disparity exists among epidemiological studies secondary to deciding the age limit for young stroke. Some studies consider <45 years as a young stroke, while some studies consider <65 years of age as a young stroke [6]. As per Global Burden of Disease 2013, the global prevalence of ischemic stroke for the age group 20–64 years was 7258,21, and hemorrhagic stroke was 3,725,085 cases respectively [1]. Black and Hispanic populations are at higher risk of stroke as compared with white populations in the United States, secondary to higher conventional risk factors [6]. Studies from Europe and the USA showed a higher incidence of stroke in women of the age group 30–44 years; however, in Chinese adults, no difference between the two genders was seen [7]. Higher mortality and recurrence of vascular events are seen more commonly in males than in females [8]. The disparities among low, middle, and high-income countries stem from genetic and cultural differences, as well as variations in access to diagnostic and therapeutic resources. Given the increasing incidence of stroke in young individuals, primary and secondary prevention should ideally begin across all income groups. Additionally, prevention strategies must be tailored to address continent and country-specific risk factors [7].

1.2 Etiology

Causes of stroke in young adults can be classified as per the trial of ORG in acute ischemic stroke (TOAST) classification used in older adults. It includes [5]:

1. Large artery atherosclerosis
   - Atherosclerotic arteriopathy.
2. Cardioembolic
   - Atrial fibrillation and other arrhythmias
   - Cardiac tumors
   - Cardiomyopathy
   - Endocarditis with or without valve vegetation
   - Patent foramen ovale (PFO) or atrial septum defect
3. Small vessel disease
   - Genetic cerebral small vessel disease-cerebral autosomal dominant arteriopathy with subcortical infarcts and leukoencephalopathy (CADASIL)

- Sporadic cerebral small vessel disease

4. Stroke of another determined cause
   - Genetics
   - Vascular
   - Drugs
   - Malignancy

5. Stroke of undetermined cause
   - Cryptogenic stroke

1.3 Large artery atherosclerosis

The conventional risk factors of stroke, including hypertension, diabetes mellitus, coronary heart disease, smoking, and heavy episodic alcohol consumption, account for almost 80% of all ischemic strokes in young adults. A deeper understanding of the impact of modifiable risk factors on the burden of stroke in young adults is crucial for developing effective preventive strategies. Research has shown that traditional stroke risk factors are more prevalent among young adults than previously believed and assumed [9]. These patients require long-term antiplatelet therapy, carotid endarterectomy, for ipsilateral carotid stenosis >50%, management of conventional risk factors, lipid-lowering agents, antihypertensives, antidiabetics, smoking cessation, etc. [5, 6].

1.4 Cardioembolic

Patients with atrial fibrillation (AF), cardiac tumors, and cardiomyopathy present with multifocal neurological symptoms with a prominent history of palpitation in patients with AF or arrhythmias. Patients with endocarditis have a history of fever, spondylodiscitis, abscess in other organs, splinter hemorrhages, and cardiac murmur. PFO or septal defects have a history of precipitation of events after Valsalva, prolonged immobility, and a history of deep venous thrombosis, with the absence of conventional risk factors. Diagnosis is confirmed with electrocardiogram (ECG), echocardiography, and transcranial Doppler bubble test for septal defects. Patients with arrhythmias and cardiomyopathy require anticoagulation for stroke prevention [10, 11]. Cardiac tumors need surgery [12]. For endocarditis patients, surgery is advised in cases of heart failure, abscess, and perforation [13]. Patients with PFO or a septal defect are given antiplatelet therapy. PFO closure is advised in recurrent PFO-related strokes [14].

1.5 Small vessel disease

CADASIL: 60–85% of patients with CADASIL present with transient ischemic attacks and ischemic strokes, with an incidence of approximately 10.4 per 100 patient-years [15]. The underlying cause remains a mutation in the NOTCH 3 gene.

Brain MRI shows white matter hyperintensity in the anterior temporal lobe or external capsule. Most events are recurrent and involve subcortical, with 67% of patients presenting with lacunar syndrome. Other clinical symptoms include psychiatric manifestations, headache, family history, and progressive cognitive impairment. These patients need long-term antiplatelet therapy [16]. However, sporadic small vessel disease occurs secondary to conventional stroke risk factors. MRI Brain shows leukoaraiosis, lacunes, microbleeds, and white matter hyperintensities.

1.6 Stroke of other determined cause

This includes an extensive list of causes, which can be divided as:

1. Genetic

   i. Autosomal dominant

   ii. Autosomal recessive

   iii. Mitochondrial

   iv. X-linked recessive

2. Vascular

3. Drugs

4. Malignancy

2. Genetic

2.1 Autosomal dominant

a. Familial Hypercholesterolemia (FH)—FH should be suspected with fasting LDL-C > 190 mg/dl in adults and > 160 mg/dl in children. FH can be established by Simon Broome's diagnostic criteria-Diagnosis of explicit FH requires [17]:

   1. Cholesterol >290 mg/dl or LDL >190 mg/dl in adults. Or Cholesterol >260 mg/dl or LDL >155 mg/dl in children <16 years of age.

   2. Tendon xanthoma in patients or a 1st or 2nd-degree relative.

   3. DNA-based on evidence of a functional LDLR, PCSK9, and apolipoprotein B (APOB) mutation.

   4. Family history of myocardial infarction before 50 years in a second-degree relative or before 60 years in a first-degree relative.

   5. Family history of raised total cholesterol >290 mg/dl in first or second-degree relative or > 260 mg/dl in sibling <16 years of age.

Definite diagnosis requires 1 and 2 or 3.

Probable diagnosis requires 1 and 4 or 1 and 5.

It affects 1/200 to 1/500 individuals worldwide. In patients with FH, those with ischemic heart disease at baseline are associated with higher ischemic stroke risk [18].

a. Ehler Danlos Syndrome (EDS) Type IV—EDS is characterized by skin hyperextensibility, joint hypermobility, and tissue fragility. There are six main types of EDS, with prominent vascular involvement occurring in type IV. There is an increased prevalence of cervical dissection, cerebral aneurysm, and cerebrovascular malformation in patients with EDS [19].

b. Marfan syndrome—An autosomal dominant disorder of connective tissue, affecting large and medium blood vessels, elastic fibers predisposing to aneurysm and dissection along with increased risk of cerebral and spinal ischemia or hemorrhage that occurs in approximately 10–20% of patients with Marfan syndrome [20].

c. Retinal vasculopathy with cerebral leukoencephalopathy (RVCL)—RVCL affecting retinal, cerebral, and systemic blood vessels occurs secondary to a frameshift mutation in the TREX1 gene. Neurological symptoms include migraine-like headaches, psychiatric disturbances, dysarthria, and hemiparesis [21]. Neuroimaging shows rim-enhancing mass lesions, punctate non-enhancing and/or nodular contrast-enhancing lesions [22]. It predominantly affects the frontal lobe and spares the corpus callosum and infratentorial tissue. Systemic manifestations are gastrointestinal bleeding, subclinical hypothyroidism, liver and renal disorders, and Raynaud's phenomenon. No therapeutic strategy is proven; however, proliferative retinopathy may respond to intravitreal bevacizumab [21].

d. COL4A mutation—COL4A mutations cause familial vasculopathy, occur on chromosome number 13, and lead to systemic small vessel disease manifestations like Raynaud's, cataracts, retinal hemorrhages, and muscle cramps. Neurological symptoms include perinatal hemorrhages, porencephaly, and infantile hemiparesis [21]. The mean age of onset is 36 years. Brain images show leukoaraiosis, microbleeds, lacunar infarcts, and dilated perivascular spaces [23].

e. Moyamoya—It is an isolated chronic, usually bilateral vasculopathy that leads to progressive narrowing of the terminal intracranial portion of the internal carotid artery (ICA) and the circle of Willis. Annual incidence is 0.5–1.5 per 1,000,000 in East Asian countries and 0.1 per 100,000 in others. In adults, it presents with hemorrhagic, and in the pediatric age group, it presents with ischemic stroke [24]. Clinical presentation includes transient ischemic attack (TIA), ischemic stroke, headache, seizures, and cognitive impairment. Lesions do not fit into a vascular territory. Conservative treatment involves aspirin, analgesics, and antiseizure medications; however, ASA 2019 guidelines recommend surgical revascularization in patients with a history of ischemic stroke or TIA [25].

2.2 Autosomal recessive

a. Deficiency of Adenosine Deaminase 2 (DADA2)—DADA2 was first described in 2014. The adenosine deaminase (ADA) enzyme occurs in two isoforms: ADA1, which is present in almost all cells and leads to severe combined immunodeficiency syndrome (SCID), and ADA2, which is present in the hematopoietic lineage. Its deficiency decreases the number of mature B cells, alters endothelial integrity, and causes chronic neutrophil activation [26].

Clinical presentation depends on the system's predominant involvement, whether vascular, immune, or hematologic, and symptoms range from fever, ischemic stroke, and portal hypertension to B-cell deficiency, pure red cell aplasia, cytopenia, or bone marrow failure, respectively. Neurological manifestations occur in approximately 51% of patients and include predominantly ischemic stroke (27%), lacunar stroke (14%), cranial nerve palsy (14%), hemorrhagic stroke (12%), and polyneuropathy (9%) [27]. Areas of stroke predilection include the brainstem, cerebellum, and deep brain nuclei [28]. Perivascular enhancement on MRI is characteristic of ADA2 deficiency [29].

High-dose systemic glucocorticoids are effective in reducing inflammation during the acute phase; however, many patients experience refractory or relapsing disease when tapering is attempted. For patients with vasculitic predominant manifestations, TNF-alpha inhibition has shown high efficacy. Anti-TNF has strong protective effects against stroke. Patients with immunodeficiency and cytopenia-driven phenotypes are less responsive to TNF-alpha inhibition, and they require hematopoietic stem cell transplantation [26].

a. CARASIL—Cerebral arteriopathy with subcortical infarcts and leukoencephalopathy has a triad of alopecia, spondylosis deformans, and cerebral small vessel disease. Premature baldness is seen in 72% of patients with CARASIL. 23% develop stroke before 40 years of age. MRI changes include bilateral periventricular subcortical white matter hyperintensity [30].

b. Anti-Phospholipid Antibody Syndrome (APAS)—The prevalence of APAS is 40–50,100,000 subjects. The presence of any antiphospholipid antibody increases the risk of cerebrovascular events by 5.48-fold for those under the age of 50 years. 30% of patients present with ischemic stroke or TIA as initial presentation [31]. The most common finding in MRI is white matter hyperintensity, cerebellar infarct, bilateral border zone infarcts, and stenotic lesions on MR angiography, mainly the bilateral internal carotid artery and M1 segment of middle cerebral artery (MCA) are seen [32]. Primary thromboprophylaxis in an antiphospholipid antibody-positive patient with low-dose aspirin was shown to reduce the risk of first thrombosis by 50% [31]. In secondary prophylaxis, long-term anticoagulation with oral anticoagulants is required [33].

c. Sickle cell disease–Ischemic or hemorrhagic stroke occurs in approximately 8% of children with sickle cell disease without treatment. Silent cerebral infarction is also common in sickle cell disease [34]. The risk of stroke is highest during the first decade and most significant between ages 2 and 5 years [35]. A child with sickle cell disease is 333 times at risk than one without [36]. Patients with abnormal velocity of intracranial blood vessels on transcranial Doppler are at increased risk of stroke, with a risk of up to 40% within 3 years [37]. The mechanism of stroke in sickle cell disease is multifactorial and includes abnormal adherence of sickled red blood cells to vascular endothelium, hemolysis-induced endothelial cell activation, a hypercoagulable state, and alteration in vasomotor tone. Red blood cell transfusion remains the most widely used preventive strategy measure for stroke these patients with sickle cell disease [38].

d. Inborn errors of metabolism—These disorders are characterized by early or premature atherosclerosis caused by a defect in lipid or amino acid metabolism, cerebrovascular occlusive disease secondary to accumulation of non-metabolized substrate, or ischemia at the molecular level [39].

e. Disorder of biolipid metabolism–Cerebrotendinous xanthomatosis (CTX) leads to bilateral cataracts, achilles tendon xanthoma, diarrhea, and dementia with stroke, mainly affecting large and small arteries and the dentate nucleus in the cerebellum. Progressive accumulation of cholestanol in the brain is the main mechanism responsible for cerebral symptoms in CTX [40]. S. Cholestanol levels and urinary bile alcohol levels are raised with low to normal serum cholesterol and low HDL [41]. MRI shows typical bilateral and symmetrical hyperintensities in the dentate nuclei [42]. A combination of chenodeoxycholic acid and simvastatin is effective in reducing further serum cholestanol and the progression of the disease [43]. Tangier disease is an extremely rare condition causing neuropathy, premature atherosclerosis, and enlarged orange tonsils, with low levels of APOA1 and cholesterol in serum, and needs supportive treatment [44].

f. Disorder of amino and organic acid metabolism-Glutaric aciduria type I and propionic acidemia are other inborn errors of metabolisms (IEMs), mainly affecting the basal ganglia with macrocephaly, dystonia, and choreoathetosis in glutaric acidemia and pancreatitis, osteopenia, hypogammaglobulinemia, and bone marrow suppression in propionic acidemia, respectively. Management involves a diet deficient in lysine, hydroxylysine, and tryptophan, supplemented with carnitine, riboflavin, baclofen, and anticholinergics in glutaric aciduria, and restriction of natural proteins, carnitine, biotin supplementation, and alkaline therapy for chronic acidosis [39]. Deficiency of cystathionine beta-synthase or methylenetetrahydrofolate reductase (MHTFR) results in homocystinuria. Clinical manifestations involve ectopia lentis, skeletal abnormalities, and osteoporosis. A homocysteine level of more than 15 umol/L increases the ischemic stroke risk in a nonlinear association [45].

2.3 Mitochondrial disorders

MELAS—Stroke-like lesions are the hallmark of MELAS and manifest clinically as hemianopsia, hemiparesis, confusion, migraine-like headaches, vomiting, or seizures [46]. The pathophysiology of stroke-like lesions in patients with MELAS remains incompletely understood. Proposed mechanisms suggest a combination of mitochondrial cytopathy and angiopathy affecting small cerebral vessels [47]. In acute episodes, MRI shows hyperintensity in diffusion weighted images (DWI) and apparent diffusion coefficient (ADC) with hyperperfusion in perfusion weighted images (PWI) in areas outside the vascular territory [47]. There is no definitive therapy yet. L-arginine therapy can be beneficial in stroke-like episode treatment and prevention [48].

2.4 X-linked recessive

Fabry's disease is a lysosomal storage disease with a deficiency of the enzyme alpha-galactosidase. It mainly affects the vertebrobasilar circulation. Symptoms include transient ischemic attacks, vertigo, hearing impairment, tinnitus, and cognitive disturbance. Other symptoms include painful paresthesia, hypohidrosis, angiokeratoma, cardiac abnormality, cornea verticillate, proteinuria, and gut dysmotility

[49]. Fabry disease contributes to 1.2% of strokes in young patients [50]. Management involves enzyme replacement therapy [49].

3. Vascular

i. Arterial dissection—Cervical artery dissection accounts for around 20% of ischemic stroke cases in young adults. Risk factors for dissection include male gender, migraine, hyperhomocysteinemia, recent infection, trauma, and smoking [51]. Carotid artery dissection is more common than vertebral artery dissection [52]. Cervical artery dissection should be considered in a young adult with unilateral head or neck pain with neurological deficit or a risk factor for dissection. The classical appearance of cervical artery dissection on color Doppler imaging is a candle flame tapering appearance within the lumen and stenosis. The carotid string sign refers to a string of contrast material distal to the dissection in the internal carotid artery [53]. Management involves antithrombotic agents. Within 4.5 hours of onset, IV thrombolysis is safe in cervical artery dissection-related stroke [52]. There is debate about whether antiplatelet or anticoagulant agents are superior at preventing a stroke. A meta-analysis looking at 40 non-randomized trials of 1636 patients with cervical artery dissection, showed that recurrent stroke risk with antiplatelet therapy vs. anticoagulation therapy was 2.6% (13/499) and 1.8% respectively (20/1137) (odds ratio 1.49) and risk of death was 1.00% (5/499) vs. 0.8% (9/1137) (odd ratio 1.27) respectively. These differences were not significant [53]. Cochrane review 2010 found no evidence for either drug in internal carotid artery dissection. As per the European Stroke Organization 2017, 6–12 months of treatment is adequate for patients where recanalization has occurred; however, in cases of residual dissecting aneurysm or stenosis, long-term antiplatelets are recommended. Both the European Stroke Organization and the American Stroke Association guidelines recommend considering endovascular therapy in those patients with recurrent ischemic events despite the best medical treatment.

ii. Vasculitis—Vasculitis increases the ischemic stroke risk by affecting vessel lumina and causing distal tissue ischemia. It also increases the stroke risk by affecting the vessel wall integrity. The site and size of the stroke depend on the vessel involved, whether the large or small vessel is involved. Large and medium vessels are typically involved in Takayasu arteritis, Polyarteritis nodosa, Kawasaki disease, respectively, and present with the sudden onset of contralateral hemiparesis. Small vessel lesions in ANCA-associated, cryoglobulinemic, and Eosinophilic granulomatous polyangiitis result in subacute, non-localizing complaints like headaches, seizures, cognitive decline, and behavioral changes [54]. On the other hand, primary angiitis of central nervous system (CNS) (PACNS) can also cause headache, cognitive deficits, and focal neurological deficits. The average affected age group is 42 years (24–63 years). Management of vasculitis, whether systemic or CNS vasculitis, is systemic steroid pulse with long-term immunomodulation [55].

iii. Migraine—Migrainous infarction is seen commonly in females suffering from migraine with aura and mainly involves the posterior circulation territory. Various factor contributes to stroke in migraine-like cortical spreading depression that leads to a change in flow dynamics, increasing vascular resistance. Increased inflammation, endothelial dysfunction, and genetics all contribute to stroke pathogenesis in migraine. Currently, there are no recommended guidelines for primary prophylaxis of stroke in migraine [56]. Young females with migraine with aura should also avoid oral contraception as it increases the stroke risk in these females [57].

iv. Reversible cerebral vasoconstriction syndrome (RCVS)—Patient presents with thunderclap headaches lasting 1–3 hours, with or without focal neurological symptoms or seizures. Angiography shows segmental narrowing of the branches of cerebral arteries. Management includes eliminating precipitating events and blood pressure control. The main diagnostic criteria of RCVS by Calabrese et al. [58].

v. Conventional angiography magnetic resonance angiography (MRA) showing widespread segmental cerebral artery vasoconstriction ("string and beads")

vi. No evidence of an aneurysmal subarachnoid hemorrhage

vii. Normal or almost normal cerebrospinal fluid analysis

viii. Acute and severe headache, with or without focal neurological deficits

ix. Reversibility of angiographic abnormalities within 3 months.

x. Various precipitating factors include drug, pregnancy, preeclampsia, eclampsia, pheochromocytoma, neuroendocrine tumor, traumatic brain injury, porphyria, unruptured cerebral aneurysm, or idiopathic [59]. Management involves nimodipine for headache and blood pressure monitoring. For prophylaxis, patients are advised to avoid the precipitating factors [60].

4. Drugs

Drug abuse is a common cause of stroke in young adults, with psychomotor stimulants like amphetamine and cocaine being the most frequently implicated. Less commonly, opioids and psychomimetics like cannabis are also associated with stroke. Toxicology screening should be conducted in all suspected cases [61]. Anabolic steroid use is associated with cerebral venous thrombosis, and heroin abuse is related to hemorrhagic stroke. Patients with tramadol, cannabis, and cocaine use disorders are more likely to experience strokes in the posterior than in the anterior circulation. Additionally, individuals with heroin use disorders had significantly higher mortality rates than those without heroin use disorders [62].

5. Malignancy

Patients with newly diagnosed cancer have an increased risk of both ischemic and hemorrhagic stroke, with 5–10% of stroke patients having active cancer. The most identified malignancies include hematologic cancers, long digestive tract cancer, lung cancer, and pancreatic cancer. The mechanism remains in a hypercoagulable state, with direct tumor effects, infections, and therapies involved in treatment. Acute treatment with IV thrombolysis is beneficial in patients with nonmetastatic disease. Prognosis is worse in patients than in patients without cancer [63].

1. Stroke of undetermined cause—In these cases, no cause or attributable risk factors are identified after thorough investigations. They are treated with conventional long-term antiplatelet therapy. The definition of embolic stroke of the unknown source is based on the exclusion of lacunar infarction by brain imaging, arterial stenosis of more than 50% or dissection of the respective brain supplying artery by angiography or ultrasound, atrial fibrillation by at least 24-hour ECG monitoring, as well as some rare causes [64].

2. Stroke associated with pregnancy—Stroke in young females deserves special mention separately. The incidence of stroke in a pregnant female is three times higher than in a nonpregnant female of similar age. Half of the maternal strokes are hemorrhagic, contrary to the general population, where 87% of strokes are ischemic [65]. Many conditions associated with pregnancy contribute to the risk of stroke and include thrombophilia, heart disease/peripartum cardiomyopathy, migraine, lupus, hypertensive disorder of pregnancy, thrombocytopenia, and gestational diabetes [66]. The highest risk of maternal stroke occurs in the peripartum and immediate postpartum period up to 2 weeks after delivery [65].

Posterior reversible encephalopathy syndrome (PRES) and reversible cerebrovascular vasoconstriction syndrome (RCVS) are commonly seen in patients with preeclampsia and occur secondary to endothelial dysfunction, inflammation, and sympathetic hyperactivity [67]. Cerebral venous thrombosis is one of the most common cerebrovascular complications in pregnancy, affecting approximately 11.6 per 100,000 deliveries [68]. Females diagnosed with moyamoya during pregnancy two-thirds present with hemorrhagic stroke with high maternal and fetal morbidity and mortality [69].

Women with antiphospholipid syndrome, lupus, or other autoimmune disorders are considered high risk and should be started on aspirin after 12 weeks of pregnancy for preeclampsia prevention [70]. These maternal strokes could be avoided with targeted prevention efforts and early recognition of warning signs, and require close collaboration between both neurologists and obstetricians.

6. Conclusion

Stroke in young adults is rising globally. Apart from conventional risk factors, genetic and region-specific risk factors play an important role. Early measures as primary prevention can substantially reduce the burden of stroke and improve the quality of life of young individuals, as stroke patients have to deal with psychosocial consequences as well after a stroke. There is a need for studies on young stroke prevalence and causes from different countries, as different regions affect the genetics and environmental factors contributing to stroke.

Conflict of interest

The author declares no conflict of interest.

DOI: http://dx.doi.org/10.5772/intechopen.1010174

Author details

Neetika Sharma* and Ashish Sharma
Department of Neurology, AIIMS, Bilaspur, H.P., India

*Address all correspondence to: sharmadrneetika@gmail.com

References

[1] Krishnamurthi RV, Moran AE, Feigin VL, Barker-Collo S, Norrving B, Mensah GA, et al. Stroke prevalence, mortality and disability-adjusted life years in adults aged 20-64 years in 1990-2013: Data from the global burden of disease 2013 study. Neuroepidemiology. 2015;**45**(3):190-202

[2] Bukhari S, Yaghi S, Bashir Z. Stroke in young adults. Journal of Clinical Medicine. 2023;**12**(15):4999

[3] Bejot Y, Daubail B, Jacquin A, Durier J, Osseby GV, Rouaud O, et al. Trends in the incidence of ischaemic stroke in young adults between 1985 and 2011: The Dijon stroke registry. Journal of Neurology, Neurosurgery, and Psychiatry. 2014;**85**(5):509-513

[4] Madsen TE, Khoury JC, Leppert M, Alwell K, Moomaw CJ, Sucharew H, et al. Temporal trends in stroke incidence over time by sex and age in the GCNKSS. Stroke. 2020;**51**(4):1070-1076

[5] Ekker MS, Boot EM, Singhal AB, Tan KS, Debette S, Tuladhar AM, et al. Epidemiology, aetiology, and management of ischaemic stroke in young adults. Lancet Neurology. 2018;**17**(9):790-801

[6] Hathidara MY, Saini V, Malik AM. Stroke in the young: A global update. Current Neurology and Neuroscience Reports. 2019;**19**(11):91

[7] Boot E, Ekker MS, Putaala J, Kittner S, De Leeuw FE, Tuladhar AM. Ischaemic stroke in young adults: A global perspective. Journal of Neurology, Neurosurgery, and Psychiatry. 2020;**91**(4):411-417

[8] Rutten-Jacobs LCA, Arntz RM, Maaijwee NAM, Schoonderwaldt HC, Dorresteijn LD, Van Dijk EJ, et al. Long-term mortality after stroke among adults aged 18 to 50 years. Journal of the American Medical Association. 2013;**309**(11):1136

[9] Aigner A, Grittner U, Rolfs A, Norrving B, Siegerink B, Busch MA. Contribution of established stroke risk factors to the burden of stroke in young adults. Stroke. 2017;**48**(7):1744-1751

[10] European Stroke Organisation (ESO) Executive Committee; ESO Writing Committee. Guidelines for management of ischaemic stroke and transient ischaemic attack 2008. Cerebrovascular Diseases. 2008;**25**(5):457-507. DOI: 10.1159/000131083. Epub 2008 May 6. PMID: 18477843

[11] Kernan WN, Ovbiagele B, Black HR, Bravata DM, Chimowitz MI, Ezekowitz MD, et al. Guidelines for the prevention of stroke in patients with stroke and transient ischemic attack: A guideline for healthcare professionals from the American Heart Association/ American Stroke Association. Stroke. 2014;**45**(7):2160-2236

[12] Abu Abeeleh M, Saleh S, Alhaddad E, Alsmady M, Alshehabat M, Bani Ismail Z, et al. Cardiac myxoma: Clinical characteristics, surgical intervention, intra-operative challenges and outcome. Perfusion. 2017;**32**(8):686-690

[13] Prendergast BD, Tornos P. Surgery for infective endocarditis: Who and when? Circulation. 2010;**121**(9):1141-1152

[14] Ando T, Holmes AA, Pahuja M, Javed A, Briasoulis A, Telila T, et al. Meta-analysis comparing patent foramen Ovale closure versus medical therapy to prevent recurrent cryptogenic stroke.

The American Journal of Cardiology. 2018;**121**(5):649-655

[15] Peters N, Herzog J, Opherk C, Dichgans M. A two-year clinical follow-up study in 80 CADASIL subjects: Progression patterns and implications for clinical trials. Stroke. 2004;**35**(7):1603-1608

[16] Chabriat H, Joutel A, Dichgans M, Tournier-Lasserve E, Bousser MG. CADASIL. Lancet Neurology. 2009;**8**(7):643-653

[17] Singh S, Bittner V. Familial hypercholesterolemia—Epidemiology, diagnosis, and screening. Current Atherosclerosis Reports. 2015;**17**(2):3

[18] Hovland A, Mundal LJ, Igland J, Veierød MB, Holven KB, Bogsrud MP, et al. Risk of ischemic stroke and Total cerebrovascular disease in familial hypercholesterolemia: A register study from Norway. Stroke. 2019;**50**(1):172-174

[19] Kim ST, Cloft H, Flemming KD, Kallmes DF, Lanzino G, Brinjikji W. Increased prevalence of cerebrovascular disease in hospitalized patients with Ehlers-Danlos syndrome. Journal of Stroke and Cerebrovascular Diseases. 2017;**26**(8):1678-1682

[20] WitykRJ,ZanferrariC,OppenheimerS. Neurovascular complications of Marfan syndrome: A retrospective, hospital-based study. Stroke. 2002;**33**(3):680-684

[21] Søndergaard CB, Nielsen JE, Hansen CK, Christensen H. Hereditary cerebral small vessel disease and stroke. Clinical Neurology and Neurosurgery. 2017;**155**:45-57

[22] Stam AH, Kothari PH, Shaikh A, Gschwendter A, Jen JC, Hodgkinson S, et al. Retinal vasculopathy with cerebral leukoencephalopathy and systemic manifestations. Brain. 2016;**139**(11): 2909-2922

[23] Lanfranconi S, Markus HS. *COL4A1* mutations as a monogenic cause of cerebral small vessel disease: A systematic review. Stroke. Aug 2010;**41**(8):e513-8. DOI: 10.1161/STROKEAHA.110.581918. Epub 2010 Jun 17. PMID: 20558831

[24] Ihara M, Yamamoto Y, Hattori Y, Liu W, Kobayashi H, Ishiyama H, et al. Moyamoya disease: Diagnosis and interventions. Lancet Neurology. 2022;**21**(8):747-758

[25] Rupareliya C, Lui F. Moyamoya disease. In: StatPearls [Internet]. Treasure Island (FL): StatPearls Publishing; 2024. Available from: http://www.ncbi.nlm.nih.gov/books/NBK535455/ [Accessed: January 6, 2025]

[26] Kendall JL, Springer JM. The many faces of a monogenic autoinflammatory disease: Adenosine deaminase 2 deficiency. Current Rheumatology Reports. 2020;**22**(10):64

[27] Meyts I, Aksentijevich I. Deficiency of adenosine deaminase 2 (DADA2): Updates on the phenotype, genetics, pathogenesis, and treatment. Journal of Clinical Immunology. 2018;**38**(5):569-578

[28] Barron KS, Aksentijevich I, Deuitch NT, Stone DL, Hoffmann P, Videgar-Laird R, et al. The Spectrum of the deficiency of adenosine deaminase 2: An observational analysis of a 60 patient cohort. Frontiers in Immunology. 2022;**12**:811473

[29] Geraldo AF, Caorsi R, Tortora D, Gandolfo C, Ammendola R, Alessio M, et al. Widening the neuroimaging features of adenosine

deaminase 2 deficiency. American Journal of Neuroradiology. 2021;**42**(5):975-979

[30] Khandelwal D, Mathur V, Vyas A, Ghunawat J, Bagaria AK. CARASIL – A review of patients from India. Neurology India. 2021;**69**(5):1359-1362

[31] Žigon P, editor. Antiphospholipid Syndrome - Recent Advances in Clinical and Basic Aspects [Internet]. London, UK: IntechOpen; 2022. Available from: https://www.intechopen.com/books/10322 [Accessed: January 8, 2025]

[32] Kaichi Y, Kakeda S, Moriya J, Ohnari N, Saito K, Tanaka Y, et al. Brain MR findings in patients with systemic lupus erythematosus with and without antiphospholipid antibody syndrome. American Journal of Neuroradiology. 2014;**35**(1):100-105

[33] Khamashta M, Taraborelli M, Sciascia S, Tincani A. Antiphospholipid syndrome. Best Practice & Research. Clinical Rheumatology. 2016;**30**(1):133-148

[34] Hirtz D, Kirkham FJ. Sickle cell disease and stroke. Pediatric Neurology. 2019;**95**:34-41

[35] Ohene-Frempong K, Weiner SJ, Sleeper LA, Miller ST, Embury S, Moohr JW, et al. Cerebrovascular accidents in sickle cell disease: Rates and risk factors. Blood. 1998;**91**(1):288-294

[36] Broderick J, Talbot GT, Prenger E, Leach A, Brott T. Stroke in children within a major metropolitan area: The surprising importance of intracerebral Hemorrhage. Journal of Child Neurology. 1993;**8**(3):250-255

[37] Verduzco LA, Nathan DG. Sickle cell disease and stroke. Blood. 2009;**114**(25):5117-5125

[38] Switzer JA, Hess DC, Nichols FT, Adams RJ. Pathophysiology and treatment of stroke in sickle-cell disease: Present and future. Lancet Neurology. 2006;**5**(6):501-512

[39] Kalidas K, Behrouz R. Inherited metabolic disorders and cerebral infarction. Expert Review of Neurotherapeutics. 2008;**8**(11): 1731-1741

[40] Ute P, Ulla A, Magnus H, Wolfgang S, Steve M, Ingemar B. On the mechanism of cerebral accumulation of cholestanol in patients with cerebrotendinous xanthomatosis. Journal of Lipid Research. 2007;**48**(5):1167-1174

[41] Muhammed K, Nandakumar G, Saritha S. Cerebrotendinous xanthomatosis: Need for early diagnosis. Indian Journal of Dermatology, Venereology and Leprology. 2006;**72**(5):364

[42] De Stefano N, Dotti MT, Mortilla M, Federico A. Magnetic resonance imaging and spectroscopic changes in brains of patients with cerebrotendinous xanthomatosis. Brain. 2001;**124**(1):121-131

[43] Verrips A, Wevers RA, Van Engelen BGM, Keyser A, Wolthers BG, Barkhof F, et al. Effect of simvastatin in addition to chenodeoxycholic acid in patients with cerebrotendinous xanthomatosis. Metabolism. 1999;**48**(2):233-238

[44] Sinha S. Tangier disease--a diagnostic challenge in countries endemic for leprosy. Journal of Neurology, Neurosurgery, and Psychiatry. 2004;**75**(2):301-304

[45] Holmen M, Hvas AM, Arendt JFH. Hyperhomocysteinemia and ischemic stroke: A potential dose-response association-a systematic review and

meta-analysis. TH Open : Companion Journal to Thrombosis and Haemostasis. 2021;**5**(3):e420-e437

[46] Finsterer J, Wakil SM. Stroke-like episodes, peri-episodic seizures, and MELAS mutations. European Journal of Paediatric Neurology. 2016;**20**(6):824-829

[47] Gramegna LL, Cortesi I, Mitolo M, Evangelisti S, Talozzi L, Cirillo L, et al. Major cerebral vessels involvement in patients with MELAS syndrome: Worth a scan? A systematic review. Journal of Neuroradiology. 2021;**48**(5):359-366

[48] Koga Y, Povalko N, Inoue E, Nakamura H, Ishii A, Suzuki Y, et al. Therapeutic regimen of l-arginine for MELAS: 9-year, prospective, multicenter, clinical research. Journal of Neurology. 2018;**265**(12):2861-2874

[49] Barrett KM, Meschia JF. Genetic stroke syndromes. Continuum: Lifelong Learning in Neurology. 2014;**20**:399-411

[50] Rolfs A, Böttcher T, Zschiesche M, Morris P, Winchester B, Bauer P, et al. Prevalence of Fabry disease in patients with cryptogenic stroke: A prospective study. The Lancet. 2005;**366**(9499):1794-1796

[51] Jazbec L, Menih M, Arh R. Ischemic stroke in young adults caused by cervical artery dissection—A retrospective study. International Journal of Angiology. 2022;**31**(02):126-130

[52] Lee VH, Brown RD, Mandrekar JN, Mokri B. Incidence and outcome of cervical artery dissection: A population-based study. Neurology. 2006;**67**(10):1809-1812

[53] Clark M, Unnam S, Ghosh S. A review of carotid and vertebral artery dissection. British Journal of Hospital Medicine. 2022;**83**(4):1-11

[54] Younger DS. Stroke due to Vasculitis in children and adults. Neurologic Clinics. 2019;**37**(2):279-302

[55] Beuker C, Strunk D, Rawal R, Schmidt-Pogoda A, Werring N, Milles L, et al. Primary Angiitis of the CNS: A systematic review and meta-analysis. Neurology Neuroimmunology and Neuroinflammation. 2021;**8**(6):e1093

[56] Zhang Y, Parikh A, Qian S. Migraine and stroke. Stroke and Vascular Neurology. 2017;**2**(3):160-167

[57] MacClellan LR, Giles W, Cole J, Wozniak M, Stern B, Mitchell BD, et al. Probable migraine with visual Aura and Risk of ischemic stroke: The stroke prevention in young women study. Stroke. 2007;**38**(9):2438-2445

[58] Calabrese LH, Dodick DW, Schwedt TJ, Singhal AB. Narrative review: Reversible cerebral vasoconstriction syndromes. Annals of Internal Medicine. 2007;**146**(1):34

[59] Erhart DK, Ludolph AC, Althaus K. RCVS: By clinicians for clinicians—A narrative review. Journal of Neurology. 2023;**270**(2):673-688

[60] Chen SP, Fuh JL, Wang SJ. Reversible cerebral vasoconstriction syndrome: An under-recognized clinical emergency. Therapeutic Advances in Neurological Disorders. 2010;**3**(3):161-171

[61] Fonseca AC, Ferro JM. Drug abuse and stroke. Current Neurology and Neuroscience Reports. 2013;**13**(2):325

[62] Rizk HI, Magdy R, Emam K, Mohammed MS, Aboulfotooh AM. Substance use disorder in young adults with stroke: Clinical characteristics and outcome. Acta Neurologica Belgica. 2024;**124**(1):65-72

[63] Zuber M. Stroke and cancer. Revue Neurologique (Paris). 2023;**179**(5): 417-424

[64] Weimar C. Stroke of undetermined cause: Workup and secondary prevention. Current Opinion in Neurology. 2016;**29**(1):4-8

[65] Miller EC. Maternal stroke associated with pregnancy. Continuum: Lifelong Learning in Neurology. 2022;**28**(1):93-121

[66] Camargo EC, Singhal AB. Stroke in pregnancy: A multidisciplinary approach. Obstetrics and Gynecology Clinics of North America. 2021;**48**(1):75-96

[67] McDermott M, Miller EC, Rundek T, Hurn PD, Bushnell CD. Preeclampsia: Association with posterior reversible encephalopathy syndrome and stroke. Stroke. 2018;**49**(3):524-530

[68] Sells C, Feske S. Stroke in pregnancy. Seminars in Neurology. 2017;**37**(06):669-678

[69] Maragkos GA, Ascanio LC, Chida K, Boone MD, Ogilvy CS, Thomas AJ, et al. Moyamoya disease in pregnancy: A systematic review. Acta Neurochirurgica. 2018;**160**(9):1711-1719

[70] Gestational Hypertension and Preeclampsia. ACOG practice bulletin, number 222. Obstetrics and Gynecology. 2020;**135**(6):e237-e260

Chapter 5

Risk Factors and Management of Stroke in Young Adults

Rajeshwar Sahonta and Anusha Thomas

Abstract

Stroke is traditionally associated with older populations, but its rising incidence among younger adults presents significant clinical and socioeconomic challenges. This paper explores the epidemiology, risk factors, and consequences of stroke in young individuals, defined as those under 45 years. Unlike older adults, young stroke patients exhibit a more heterogeneous risk factor profile, including genetic predisposition, lifestyle influences, and rare vascular disorders. The study underscores the urgent need for early identification, preventive strategies, and targeted interventions to mitigate long-term morbidity and economic burden. Understanding modifiable and non-modifiable risk factors is essential for developing comprehensive stroke prevention frameworks tailored to younger populations.

Keywords: young stroke, epidemiology, risk factor, prevention, neurology, socioeconomic impact

1. Introduction

Stroke bears a vast neurological disease burden, as evidenced by emerging and expansive epidemiological literature. Stroke is the second most frequent cause of death worldwide, after ischemic heart disease, and the third leading cause of disability. While a specific definition of "young stroke" is lacking, the vast majority of authors consider "young stroke" to pertain to individuals under 45 years of age [1]. Younger stroke patients tend to have better short-term outcomes, as evidenced by a higher percentage (60%) achieving a modified Rankin Scale (mRS) score of 0–2 at 28 days post-stroke compared to older patients (46%). However, for younger patients, long-term prognosis remains a crucial area of focus, as they will live longer with the consequences of stroke. Rapid identification of causes and risk factors of ischemic stroke in young adults is key to optimizing treatment and preventing recurrence [2].

2. Incidence and epidemiology

The prevalence of stroke in young adults is estimated to be about 10–14% of all strokes [3]. From 1990 to 2013, there was an observed rise in the prevalence of stroke cases, deaths, and disability-adjusted life years (DALYs) among adults aged 20–64 years. Developing countries saw a 36.7% increase in stroke-related deaths

(95% uncertainty intervals 26.3–48.5) in this age group, while developed countries experienced a decline in these trends [4]. In the U.S., individuals aged 20–44 account for 10–15% of all strokes [5], with ischemic strokes comprising 65%, intracerebral hemorrhages 17%, and subarachnoid hemorrhages 16% [6]. By 2050, it is projected that nearly half of the stroke-related expenses in the USA, including treatment, rehabilitation, and lost productivity, could be attributed to young individuals who experience a stroke [7].

3. Non-modifiable risk factors

3.1 Gender

Gender plays a role in stroke risk, with certain factors being unique or more prevalent in women. These include the use of estrogen-containing birth control, pregnancy, and migraine with aura. When all three—migraine with aura, combined oral contraceptive use, and tobacco consumption—are present, the risk of stroke is about nine times higher compared to women without these factors [8].

3.1.1 Migraine

Migraine is the most common symptom of around 80% of females. Migraines affect 91% of men and 96% of women, with 1-year prevalence rates of 6% in men and 18% in women. Ischemic stroke in younger women with migraine with aura is more prevalent among those who are less likely to have typical cardiovascular risk factors, such as hypertension, diabetes, or high cholesterol [9].

3.1.2 Pregnancy

Pregnancy—stroke is higher during the peripartum and postpartum periods compared to the antepartum period [10, 13]. Although stroke risk is generally low among young women, pregnancy, especially during the peripartum period, increases this risk [10]. Stroke events are more common during the delivery (41%) and postpartum (48%) periods than in the antepartum period (11%). The incidence of pregnancy-related strokes, including both ischemic and hemorrhagic subtypes, is estimated at approximately 34 per 100,000 pregnancies [11]. Pathways leading to hemodynamic changes and hypercoagulable states in pregnancy are shown in **Figure 1** and **Figure 2**, respectively.

Immune system: an excessive inflammatory response resulting from dysregulation of this immunomodulatory process can lead to endothelial dysfunction, a key factor in the development of preterm birth and preeclampsia and may also elevate the risk of stroke [12].

3.1.3 Exogenous estrogen

Exogenous estrogen is linked to a higher risk of stroke. Women who currently use oral contraceptive pills (OCPs) have a ≈ 2.4-fold higher risk of ischemic stroke [13] and a ≈ 1.4-fold higher risk of hemorrhagic stroke [14], according to earlier meta-analyses.

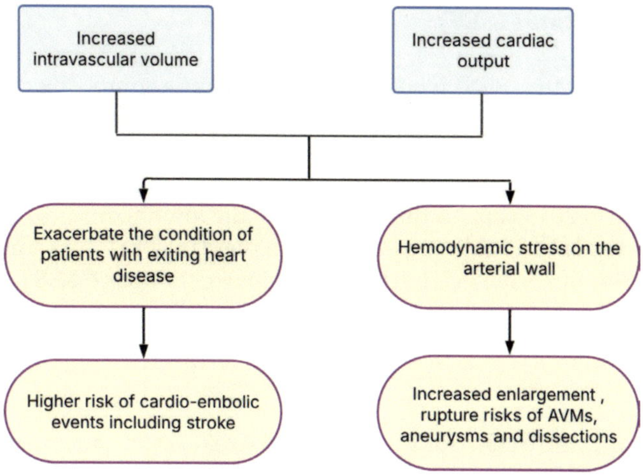

Figure 1.
Hemodynamic changes in pregnancy. AVM: arteriovenous malformations.

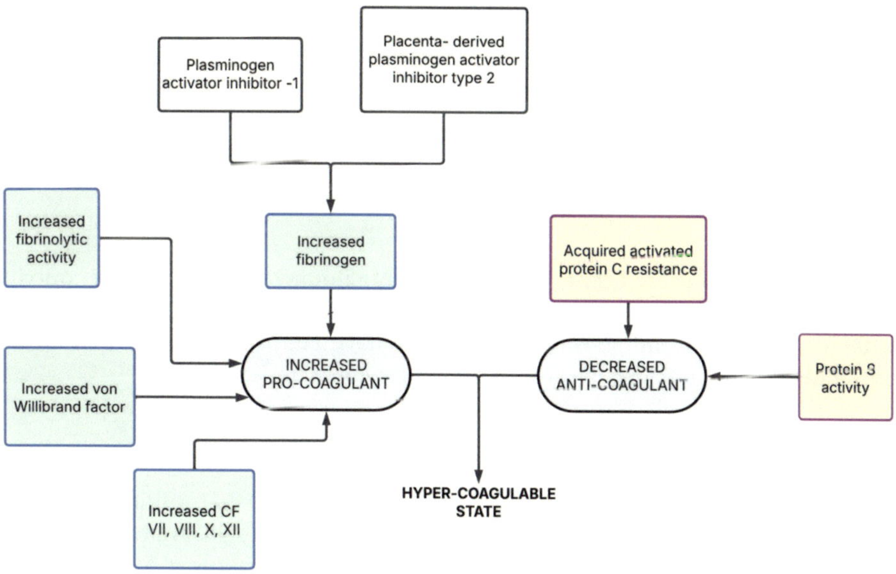

Figure 2.
Pathway leading to hyper-coagulable state in pregnancy. CF: clotting factors.

3.2 Race and ethnicity

Not every group is affected by stroke in the same way. Young non-Hispanic Black people in the United States have a stroke rate that is more than twice as high as that of White people, with fatality rates that are 36–48% higher [15]. The margin has varied over time, closing between 2008 and 2012 and then expanding once more between 2012 and 2017 [16].

3.3 Socioeconomic status (SES)

Socioeconomic status (SES) is commonly defined as a composite measure encompassing income, education, employment, and social status. Those with lower SES also tend to have worse survival outcomes and greater stroke severity compared to those with higher SES [17]. According to World Bank criteria, the age-standardized stroke-related death rate in 2019 was 3.6 times greater in the low-income group than in the high-income group [18]. Childhood exposure to the stroke belt was similarly linked to an increased risk of stroke in adulthood, and lower childhood SES had an independent effect on adult stroke risk [16].

3.4 Genetics

Genetics significantly contribute to ischemic stroke, especially in younger patients, with heritability estimates ranging from 16% to 40% depending on subtype [19, 20]. A positive family history increases stroke risk by 30–76%, with the highest genetic influence in large-vessel stroke (40%), followed by cardioembolic (33%) and small vessel disease (16%). The association between family history and stroke is strongest in the youngest group (15–24 years) [19]. Monogenic disorders, though accounting for ~5% of cases, may be underdiagnosed due to phenotypic variability and complexity [20].

4. Modifiable risk factors

4.1 Lifestyle

Changes in lifestyle are becoming more widely acknowledged as a major contributing factor to the rising number of strokes among younger people. Smoking, heavy alcohol use, poor diet, and physical inactivity all have a detrimental effect on cardiovascular health and increase the risk of stroke in people under 50.

4.1.1 Tobacco

Tobacco use was responsible for 229.77 million DALYs and 8.71 million deaths globally in 2019 [21]. The risk of stroke is increased by early exposure to tobacco smoke, including mother smoking during pregnancy and smoking at any age, with the risk increasing with younger initiation of smoking [22]. For every five extra cigarettes smoked each day, the risk of stroke rose by 12% [23]. **Figure 3** illustrates the mechanisms underlying smoke-induced thrombotic states [24, 25].

4.1.2 Alcohol

Moderate-to-heavy alcohol use increases the risk of hemorrhagic stroke, especially in young adults, and is a significant modifiable stroke risk factor [26]. Alcohol regularly causes cerebral vasospasm and elevated blood pressure, which increases the risk of ischemic stroke and atrial fibrillation. Furthermore, alcohol might exacerbate hemorrhagic stroke without causing it due to its effects on platelet activity and coagulant insufficiency [27].

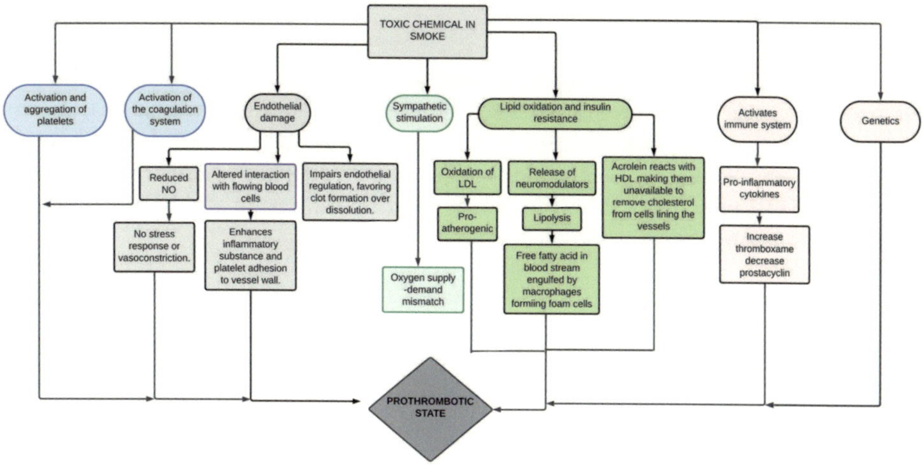

Figure 3.
Mechanism of smoke-induced prothrombotic states. NO: nitric oxide; LDL: low-density lipids.

4.1.3 Obesity and physical inactivity

Adolescent physical inactivity feeds the cycle of decreased activity and fat buildup, which leads to adult obesity, particularly abdominal obesity [28]. Thirty-one percent of people worldwide do not engage in physical activity. People who are moderately active are 20% less likely to have a stroke, and people who are very active are 27% less likely to have an ischemic or hemorrhagic stroke [29].

4.1.4 Illicit drug abuse

Drug users under the age of 35 are 6.5 times more likely to have a stroke than non-users, and cerebrovascular problems, in addition to overdose, suicide, and violence, contribute to morbidity. The primary illegal substances associated with stroke include cocaine, amphetamines, ecstasy, heroin/opiates, phencyclidine, lysergic acid diethylamide, and cannabis [30].

4.1.4.1 Cocaine

Cocaine-induced vasospasm is multifactorial, influencing calcium channels, raising catecholamine levels, and boosting endothelin-1, which results in vasoconstriction and endothelial damage [30]. It increases the generation of thromboxane and the formation of thrombus by improving the platelets' reaction to arachidonic acid [31].

4.1.4.2 Amphetamine

Amphetamine dramatically increases the risk of hemorrhagic stroke in people between the ages of 18 and 44. The medication's sympathomimetic actions can result in tachycardia and temporary hypertension, which can contribute to cerebral hemorrhage even in the absence of preexisting [32].

4.1.4.3 Ecstasy

Ischemic stroke in the globus pallidus and occipital cortex can result from vasospasm and necrosis in these regions [33]. Aneurysmal dilatation, thrombosis, vascular damage, and an elevated risk of acute ischemic stroke, ICH, or subarachnoid hemorrhage (SAH) are all consequences of long-term use. Additionally, it decreases serotonin availability, which increases the risk of cerebral infarction and ICH, particularly when hypertension is present [30].

4.1.4.4 Opium

Opium readily penetrates the blood-brain barrier, producing a "rush" at injection that is followed by drowsiness. The likelihood of right-to-left pulmonary shunts and pulmonary hypertension is increased by heroin-associated strokes, which are frequently caused by cardioembolism from infective endocarditis or embolic illness from foreign particles such as starch or talcum powder. Hypotension, hypoxemia, and overdose-induced hypoxic-ischemic damage are further concerns [30].

4.2 Cardiovascular risks

4.2.1 Hypertension

Several processes that contribute to both ischemia and hemorrhagic events are involved in the pathophysiology of stroke associated with hypertension. High intraluminal pressure causes endothelial damage, which increases the permeability of the blood-brain barrier, causes cerebral edema, and facilitates ischemic lesions and thrombus development. Lacunar infarcts result from minor artery stenosis and blockage caused by the buildup of fibrinoid necrosis [34].

Chronic hypertension raises the likelihood of rupture, particularly at bifurcations, by causing arteriolar abnormalities such as fibrinoid necrosis, lipohyalinosis, medial degeneration, and microaneurysm development [35]. Vulnerable capillaries and arterioles can be ruptured by sudden increases in blood pressure. Hypertension hinders endothelium-dependent vasodilation, attenuates functional hyperemia, and decreases cerebral blood flow. Leukocyte activation and vascular inflammation are factors in the pathophysiology of stroke. A vicious cycle of hypertension and stroke risk is created when impaired arterial baroreflex sensitivity exacerbates vascular dysfunction [34].

4.2.2 Diabetes

Diabetes is an independent risk factor for stroke, linked to increased rates of ischemic strokes as opposed to hemorrhagic strokes, as well as increased morbidity and death [36]. **Figure 4** illustrates the process by which diabetes results in ischemic stroke [37, 38].

4.2.3 Dyslipidemia

Hyperlipidemia increases the risk of atherothrombotic and cardioembolic strokes and encourages coronary or cervical atherosclerosis [39]. Following a stroke, high LDL levels were linked to long-term mortality [40]. High cholesterol causes atherosclerosis, which encourages the buildup of plaque in arteries, resulting in carotid artery stenosis and raising the risk of an ischemic stroke. Chronic

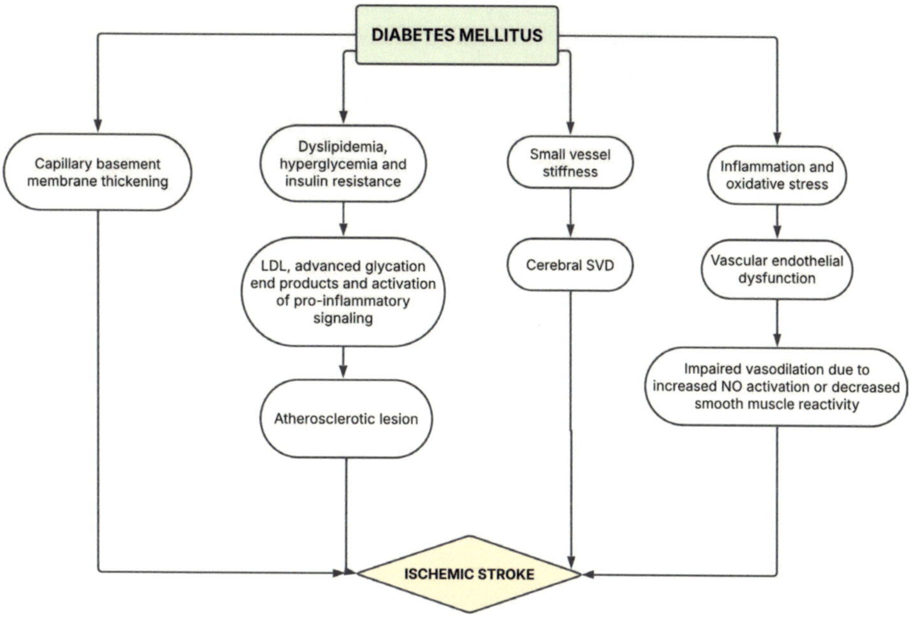

Figure 4.
Mechanism of diabetes leading to ischemic stroke. SVD: small vessel disease.

inflammation is a common feature of dyslipidemic conditions, aggravating vascular damage and promoting atherogenesis. Lipid imbalances can also affect endothelial function, making blood vessels more susceptible to thrombosis. The dyslipidemia-related prothrombotic environment further increases the risk of arterial occlusion, compounding the potential for adverse cardiovascular events [41].

4.2.4 Atrial fibrillations

Regardless of age, sex, prior myocardial infarction, or whether the AF is chronic or paroxysmal. It is linked to roughly 1 out of 6 ischemic strokes [42], with a recurrent stroke risk of up to 20% annually if treatment is not received [43]. The embolization of cardiogenic thrombi, which mainly originate from the left atrial appendage (LAA), accounts for the majority of cases [42]. Pathogenesis is depicted in **Figure 5**.

4.2.5 Cardiomyopathy

Due to an increased risk of embolism from compromised cardiac function, cardiomyopathy which includes dilated (DCM), hypertrophic (HCM), and arrhythmogenic right ventricular cardiomyopathy (ARVC), is a prominent risk factor for ischemic stroke in young people. With an incidence of 0.589 strokes per 100 person-years, HCM patients without AF are at comparable risk to those with AF [44].

4.2.6 Congenital heart disease (CHD)

About 1% of babies are born with CHD. It increases the risk of stroke, particularly in males over 40. Heart failure, diabetes, and arrhythmias are common in young individuals with CHD and stroke. According to a study conducted in Quebec, the

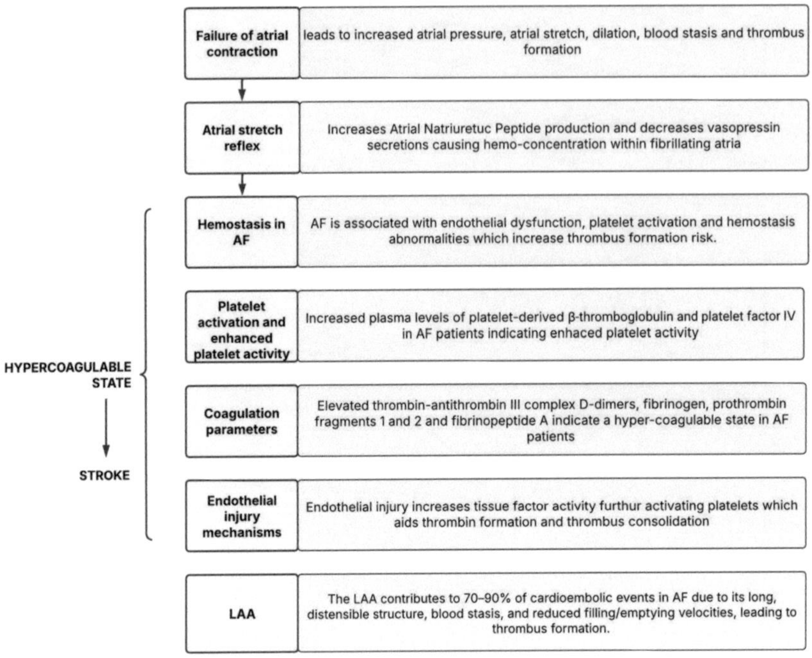

Figure 5.
Pathogenesis of stroke in atrial fibrillations. AF: atrial fibrillations; LAA: left atrial appendage.

incidence of ischemic stroke was up to 12 times higher in people aged 18 to 54 and up to 3 times higher in people aged 55 to 64 than in the general population [45].

4.2.7 Infective endocarditis

Infective endocarditis is more common in children with left-sided endocarditis and can result in stroke through embolic infarction or hemorrhage. Bacterial adherence is facilitated by the infection's disruption of the endothelium surface, which encourages turbulent blood flow and the creation of thrombotic vegetation. This risk is increased by native valve defects such as mitral valve prolapse or congenital heart disease. Once bacteria adhere, they activate immune cells and the clotting cascade, fostering vegetation growth that protects embedded bacteria [46].

5. Others

5.1 Vasculopathy, vasculitides and arteritis

5.1.1 Fabry disease (FD)

Caused by mutation in the alpha-galactosidase A gene raises the risk of stroke, especially in young men (ages 25–44), whose risk is over 12 times higher than that of the normal population. Endothelial dysfunction, cerebral hyperperfusion, prothrombosis, and increased reactive oxygen species are the main causes of vascular problems. Glycosphingolipid buildup in endothelial cells encourages the growth of smooth muscle, which raises the risk of stroke even more [47].

5.1.2 Moyamoya disease

Moyamoya disease is a rare, progressive cerebrovascular disease that is frequently associated with hereditary variables and mutations in extracellular matrix remodeling. It is characterized by artery blockage as a result of smooth muscle cell hyperplasia and luminal thrombosis. In an effort to reestablish blood flow, collateral arteries form at the base of the brain [48].

5.1.3 Takayasu arteritis

Takayasu arteritis or pulseless disease, is the chronic inflammation of the aorta and its branches, known as primarily affects females between the ages of 11 and 30. Strokes happen in 10–20% of cases, and neurological symptoms like headaches, dizziness, and transient ischemic attacks are caused by persistent ischemia caused by occlusion or stenosis of the aortic branches. Additionally, the illness may result in hypertensive crises, which could lead to hemorrhagic stroke [49].

5.1.4 MELAS (mitochondrial encephalopathy, lactic acidosis and stroke-like episodes)

MELAS (mitochondrial encephalopathy, lactic acidosis and stroke-like episodes) is a mitochondrial disease that affects 1 in 6000 people, usually under the age of 40 years. Neuroimaging reveals asymmetric lesions, and symptoms include stroke-like events, seizures, hemiplegia, cognitive impairment, and sensorineural deafness. It frequently results from a mutation in mitochondrial DNA at m.3243A > G [50], which causes cerebral edema and microangiopathy [49].

5.1.5 Fibromuscular dysplasia (FMD)

Mostly affecting women with a median age of 51.9 years, can induce stroke in younger people, especially by cervical artery dissection (CeAD), which is 70% associated with cerebral aneurysms and stroke [51].

5.1.6 Reversible cerebral vasoconstriction syndrome (RCVS)

More frequent in women peaks at age 42 and resolves in 1–3 months. It causes thunderclap headaches and sporadic neurological impairments. High blood pressure, vasoconstrictive medications, migraines, and the postpartum phase are among the triggers. Acute artery constriction is frequently normal, although imaging may reveal it. Intracerebral hemorrhage and ischemic stroke can result from RCVS [52].

5.2 Hematological conditions

5.2.1 Thrombophilic disorders

5.2.1.1 Protein C and S

Protein C and S are natural anticoagulants that prevent blood clots, raise the risk of thrombosis, including stroke, in young people. Blood tests and genetic testing for mutations in the PROC gene are used to diagnose strokes associated with this deficit, and the usual treatment is long-term anticoagulation with heparin or warfarin [53].

5.2.1.2 Deficiency in antithrombin III (AT III)

Congenital ATIII deficiency is an inherited condition that raises the risk of excessive clotting. It is a protein that prevents blood clots from forming. Low ATIII levels increase the risk of aberrant clot formation by upsetting the delicate balance between bleeding and clotting. ATIII-level blood tests are used for diagnosis, and family screening is advised. Close observation and long-term anticoagulant treatment are necessary to lower the risk of problems and deaths [54].

5.2.1.3 Factor V Leiden

Factor V mutation that prevents it from being broken down by activated protein C (APC) is the cause of this autosomal dominant genetic disorder. When factor V is still active, it promotes excessive thrombin synthesis, which results in the development of excess fibrin and clotting, mostly in veins, which can lead to diseases like pulmonary embolism and deep vein thrombosis. Although transient ischemic events are more frequent, arterial clot development that results in stroke or heart attack is uncommon [55].

5.2.1.4 Prothrombin gene 20210 G/A variant

Prothrombin gene 20210 G/A variant increases blood clotting risk and is found in about 2% of individuals of European ancestry. Recent studies, including a meta-analysis and the Genetics of Early Onset Stroke (GEOS) study, have linked this mutation to a higher risk of ischemic stroke in adults ≤55 years, particularly in younger individuals (15–42 years) [56].

5.2.1.5 Anti-phospholipid antibody syndrome

More common in younger females, is an autoimmune disease associated with venous thrombosis, usually between the ages of 30 and 40. It doubles the risk of stroke, particularly in younger patients, and affects 10–20% of people under 50 who have a stroke. It is common in patients with systemic lupus erythematosus (SLE). Stroke kills 10–15% of SLE patients, with people in their 30s to 39s having the highest risk [57].

5.2.2 Sickle cell anemia (SCA)

Sickle cell anemia (SCA) is a serious condition where stroke affects 5–10% of patients before adulthood. Elevated transcranial Doppler (TCD) velocities (>200 cm/s) significantly increase stroke risk, with children showing a 44-fold higher risk. Hydroxyurea is also known to lower stroke risk [58].

5.2.3 Hyperhomocysteinemia

Hyperhomocysteinemia is associated with thrombosis, atherosclerosis, small vessel disease, and arterial dissection. It is brought on by genetic abnormalities or deficiencies in folate, B6, and B12. It is linked to ischemic stroke and is caused by a mutation in the MTHFR gene. According to one study, young males with ischemic stroke had four times the prevalence of hyperhomocysteinemia compared to women [59, 60].

5.3 Other structural and genetic conditions

5.3.1 Carotid or vertebral artery dissection

A prominent cause of ischemic stroke in younger adults affects around 2.6 out of 100,000 persons annually, with a mean age of 45. Trauma is a common trigger; diagnostic methods include MRI, MRA, CTA, ultrasound, and angiography; dissections may have a delayed onset [60, 61].

5.3.2 Patent foramen ovale (PFO)

Patent foramen ovale (PFO) is a major cause of cryptogenic stroke, which accounts for up to 40% of strokes in young people and is present in 50% of young stroke patients under 40. The main cause of arterial stroke is paradoxical embolism, in which venous thrombi enter through the PFO. An agitated saline test and a transcranial Doppler are used to make the diagnosis. PFO closure may be taken into consideration for recurrent strokes, but antiplatelet treatment is usually used for first-time strokes [62].

6. Management

6.1 Emergency assessment

The hyperacute phase of stroke management begins immediately upon the patient's arrival at the hospital or emergency department, as shown in **Figures 6** and 7. MRI can assist in distinguishing a stroke from stroke mimics.

7. Ischemic stroke

Intravenous alteplase should be administered to young people with large strokes who qualify for thrombolysis. Ten percent of the dose should be given as a bolus over 1 minute, and the suggested dosage is 0.9 mg/kg (up to 90 mg) spread out over 60 minutes. The AHA 2019 update to the 2018 guidelines states that the normal treatment window for thrombolysis is 0–3 hours after the onset of symptoms, with an expanded window of up to 4.5 hours in some circumstances [1]. Although intravenous alteplase is the recommended treatment, patients who are eligible for mechanical thrombectomy may be evaluated for Tenecteplase (given as a single IV bolus of 0.25 mg/kg, up to 25 mg), as long as IV fibrinolysis is not contraindicated [1].

In cases of ischemic cerebral stroke, the main goal of mechanical thrombectomy (MT) is to preserve the ischemic penumbra. The following requirements for eligibility for endovascular mechanical thrombectomy therapy are outlined in the American Heart Association and American Stroke Association (AHA/ASA) recommendations for the early management of acute ischemic stroke [1, 63]: 1. A mRS

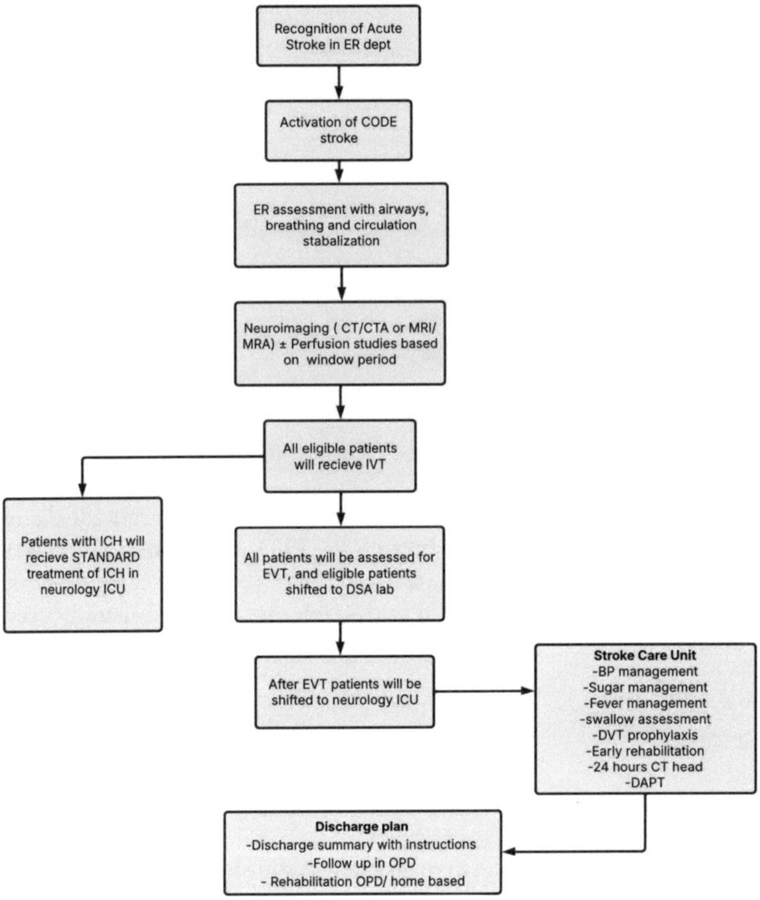

Figure 6.
Acute ishcemic stroke management. ER: emergency room; CT: computed tomography; CTA: computed tomography angiography; MRI: magnetic resonance imaging; MRA: magnetic resonance angiography; IVT: intravenous thrombolysis; ICH: intra-cranial hemorrhage; ICU: intensive care unit; EVT: endo-vascular treatment; DSA: digital subtraction angiography; DVT: deep vein thrombosis; DAPT: dual anti-platelet therapy; OPD: out patient department.

score below 2 prior to a stroke. 2. An Alberta Stroke Program Early CT Score of 6 or higher and an NIHSS of 6 or higher. 3. Within 6 hours of the commencement of symptoms, the surgery should begin. 4. The existence of a causal blockage in the proximal middle cerebral artery (M1) or internal carotid artery. 5. The patient must be at least 18 years old.

8. Intracranial hemorrhage

8.1 Hypertension management

Reducing the SBP to 140 mmHg is safe and may improve functional outcomes, per ASA guidelines. A more vigorous BP lowering with continuous intravenous infusion is necessary for SBP > 220 mmHg [64]. Drugs such as beta-blockers (labetalol, esmolol),

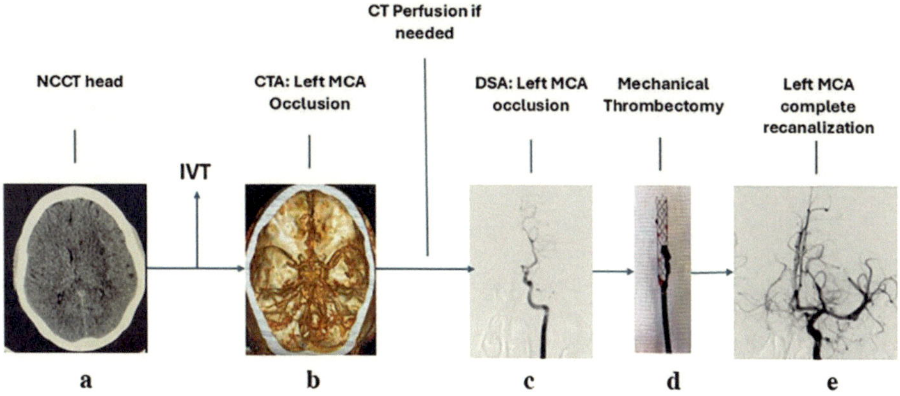

Figure 7.
Acute ischemic stroke management workflow. NCCT [a] rules out hemorrhage, followed by CTA [b] and optional CT perfusion to confirm left middle cerebral artery (MCA) occlusion. Digital subtraction angiography (DSA) [c] guides mechanical thrombectomy [d], achieving re-canalization [e], with intravenous thrombolysis (IVT) used when appropriate.

ACE inhibitors (enalapril), calcium channel blockers (nicardipine), or hydralazine should be used to progressively lower blood pressure [65].

8.2 Intracranial pressure (ICP) management

Intracranial pressure (ICP) management starts by giving osmotic agents, such as mannitol or hypertonic saline, and raising the head of the bed to 30 degrees. Typically, 1.0 to 1.5 g/kg of mannitol 20% is administered. Hyperventilation during intubation and sedation to a pCO_2 of 28–32 mmHg can be necessary if ICP increases further. In patients with a GCS <8 or indications of hydrocephalus or transtentorial herniation, the American Psychological Association advises using a parenchymal or ventricular catheter to monitor intracranial pressure (ICP) [64].

8.3 Hemostatic therapy

In patients receiving anticoagulant therapy, reversing coagulopathy is crucial. Vitamin K, prothrombin complex concentrates (PCCs), rFVIIa, and fresh frozen plasma are among the available treatment options. For thrombocytopenic patients, ASA suggests platelet concentrate; for increased INR, it suggests intravenous vitamin K with FFP or PCCs. According to the FAST study, rFVIIa decreased hematoma size but had no effect on outcomes or survival [65, 66].

9. Cardiac assessment

About 20% of strokes in young adults are cardioembolic. A 12-lead ECG is used in the initial cardiac evaluation to check for arrhythmias and prior ischemia episodes; however, it may not detect temporary arrhythmias such as paroxysmal atrial fibrillation. Implanted loop recorders can record for up to 3 years, whereas Holter monitors for 24 hours. While transesophageal echocardiogram provides superior resolution for minor diseases, transthoracic echocardiography can identify ventricular dysfunction and valvular abnormalities.

10. Patent foramen ovale (PFOs)

PFOs are present in 25% of non-stroke patients and 50% of young stroke patients [67], with the TTE bubble being a key diagnostic test [68]. Recent trials (CLOSE, REDUCE, RESPECT-PART 2) showed reduced stroke events after PFO closure [69–71].

11. Others

Diabetes, hypercholesterolemia, and blood problems can be identified with the use of basic tests such as CBC, coagulation studies, lipid profiles, and HbA1c. TSH, ESR, CRP, RPR, HIV, hemoglobin electrophoresis, toxicological screening, and pregnancy screening, when necessary, are additional tests performed on young individuals [72]. Up to 12% of strokes in young adults are caused by drug use, and excessive alcohol use is a risk factor in and of itself.

12. Stroke care unit

12.1 Glucose management

Strict glucose management (80–110 mg/dL) with insulin infusion enhances recovery in surgical critical care patients, whereas elevated entry glucose deteriorates ICH outcomes [66].

12.2 Fever management

Following an ischemic stroke, hyperthermia is prevalent, particularly when there is intraventricular bleeding, and it raises mortality. Fever duration is associated with outcomes and may be associated with the formation of hematomas in survivors who have survived for more than 72 hours [66].

12.3 DVT prophylaxis

DVT prophylaxis uses both mechanical and pharmacological techniques. Although early use of anticoagulants in ICH or massive infarctions is dangerous, they are recommended for high-risk individuals [73]. By applying pressure to the calf muscles, mechanical devices increase blood flow [74].

12.4 Swallow assessment

Pneumonia in stroke patients is frequently caused by aspiration. Screening for dysphagia on a regular basis can significantly reduce the risk of pneumonia and improve overall results [75].

13. Secondary stroke prevention

The goal of secondary prevention is to stop strokes from happening again. With a 9.4% chance at 5 years, stroke recurrence is much higher even in young stroke patients, mostly due to modifiable risk factors [76]. Before beginning antiplatelet therapy to avoid subsequent stroke, a regular non-contrast head CT scan should be performed 24 hours after treatment to check for bleeding [77].

13.1 Antiplatelet therapy

Dual antiplatelet treatment (DAPT) is recommended for strokes caused by symptomatic intracranial atherosclerosis, mild ischemic stroke (NIHSS <4), and high-risk transient ischemic attacks (TIA). To lower the incidence of recurrent stroke, DAPT is usually used for 21 days [78]. According to the 2014 American Heart Association guidelines, patients who are unable to take oral anticoagulants and have severe cerebral stenosis or ischemic stroke/TIA from atrial fibrillation should wait 90 days. Due to the possibility of bleeding, DAPT is helpful for mild strokes but not for large infarcts or severe strokes [79].

13.2 Anticoagulation

For certain stroke etiologies, anticoagulation is the recommended course of treatment. The use of anticoagulants such warfarin, apixaban, rivaroxaban, and dabigatran for cardioembolic strokes brought on by atrial fibrillation is supported by the strongest degree of evidence. Anticoagulation is also highly recommended for strokes brought on by cerebral venous sinus thrombosis. Unfractionated or low molecular weight heparin should be administered right away to patients with proven CVST, and they should then take warfarin for 3 to 6 months [80].

13.3 Addressing modifiable risk factors

For the prevention of subsequent stroke, hypertension should be controlled below 140/90 mmHg in non-diabetic patients and below 130/90 mmHg in diabetic patients [81]. A low glycemic index diet and a HgbA1C <7% are the goals of diabetes management [1]. Statins stabilize atherosclerotic plaques and manage dyslipidemia, frequently in conjunction with ezetimibe [82]. Recurrence can be avoided with lifestyle modifications like as exercise, a low salt intake, Mediterranean diets or the Dietary Approach to Stop Hypertension (DASH), and quitting smoking [83].

14. Rehabilitation post-stroke

Rehabilitation post-stroke necessitates a multidisciplinary approach since it combines medical, social, and occupational issues. Younger patients must concentrate on accepting their illness and deal with issues including adjustment and work-related stress [84].

15. Conclusion

Stroke in young adults presents a growing challenge with lifelong consequences. Early diagnosis, aggressive risk factor management, and multidisciplinary care are critical to improving outcomes. Advancements in genetics and imaging will refine treatment strategies, while public health efforts must focus on prevention and accessibility. A concerted effort is needed to reduce the burden of young stroke and enhance long-term patient support.

Abbreviations

SLE	systemic lupus erythematosus
SCA	sickle cell anemia
OCPs	oral contraceptive pills
ARVC	arrhythmogenic right ventricular cardiomyopathy
FMD	fibromuscular dysplasia
CeAD	cervical artery dissection
SVD	small vessel disease
MT	mechanical thrombectomy
AHA/ASA	The American Heart Association and American Stroke Association
MELAS	mitochondrial encephalopathy, lactic acidosis, and stroke-like episodes
CADASIL	cerebral autosomal dominant arteriopathy with subcortical infarcts and leukoencephalopathy
AIS	acute ischemic stroke
DALYs	disability-adjusted life years
ICH	intracerebral hemorrhage
mRS	modified Rankin Scale
PFO	patent foramen ovale
SVD	small vessel disease

Author details

Rajeshwar Sahonta* and Anusha Thomas
Christian Medical College, Ludhiana, India

*Address all correspondence to: sahontadr@gmail.com

References

[1] Powers WJ, Rabinstein AA, Ackerson T, Adeoye OM, Bambakidis NC, Becker K, et al. Guidelines for the early management of patients with acute ischemic stroke: 2019 update to the 2018 guidelines for the early management of acute ischemic stroke: A guideline for healthcare professionals from the American Heart Association/American Stroke Association. Stroke. 2019;**50**(12):e344-e418

[2] Nogueira RG, Jadhav AP, Haussen DC, Bonafe A, Budzik RF, Bhuva P, et al. Thrombectomy 6 to 24 hours after stroke with a mismatch between deficit and infarct. The New England Journal of Medicine. 2018;**378**(1):11-21

[3] Smajlović D. Strokes in young adults: Epidemiology and prevention. Vascular Health and Risk Management. 24 Feb 2015;**11**:157-164. DOI: 10.2147/VHRM.S53203

[4] Albers GW, Marks MP, Kemp S, Christensen S, Tsai JP, Ortega-Gutierrez S, et al. Thrombectomy for stroke at 6 to 16 hours with selection by perfusion imaging. The New England Journal of Medicine. 2018;**378**(8):708-718

[5] Maaijwee NAMM, Rutten-Jacobs LCA, Schaapsmeerders P, Van Dijk EJ, De Leeuw FE. Ischaemic stroke in young adults: Risk factors and long-term consequences. Nature Reviews. Neurology. 2014;**10**(6):315-325

[6] Kissela BM, Khoury JC, Alwell K, Moomaw CJ, Woo D, Adeoye O, et al. Age at stroke: Temporal trends in stroke incidence in a large, biracial population. Neurology. 2012;**79**(17):1781-1787

[7] Amoah D, Schmidt M, Mather C, Prior S, Herath MP, Bird ML. An international perspective on young stroke incidence and risk factors: A scoping review. BMC Public Health. 2024;**24**(1):1627

[8] Pezzini A, Grassi M, Lodigiani C, Patella R, Gandolfo C, Casoni F, et al. Pedictors of migraine subtypes in young adults with ischemic stroke: The Italian project on stroke in young adults. Stroke. 2011;**42**(1):17-21

[9] George MG. Risk factors for ischemic stroke in younger adults: A focused update. Stroke. 2020;**51**(3):729-735

[10] Ban L, Sprigg N, Abdul Sultan A, Nelson-Piercy C, Bath PM, Ludvigsson JF, et al. Incidence of first stroke in pregnant and nonpregnant women of childbearing age: A population-based cohort study from England. Journal of the American Heart Association. 2017;**6**(4):e004601

[11] Kremer C, Gdovinova Z, Bejot Y, Heldner MR, Zuurbier S, Walter S, et al. European Stroke Organisation guidelines on stroke in women: Management of menopause, pregnancy and postpartum. European Stroke Journal. 2022;**7**(2):I-XIX

[12] Yoon CW, Bushnell CD. Stroke in women: A review focused on epidemiology, risk factors, and outcomes. Journal of Stroke. 2023;**25**(1):2-15

[13] Xu Z, Li Y, Tang S, Huang X, Chen T. Current use of oral contraceptives and the risk of first-ever ischemic stroke: A meta-analysis of observational studies. Thrombosis Research. 2015;**136**(1):52-60

[14] Xu Z, Yue Y, Bai J, Shen C, Yang J, Huang X, et al. Association between oral contraceptives and risk of hemorrhagic stroke: A meta-analysis of observational

studies. Archives of Gynecology and Obstetrics. 2018;**297**(5):1181-1191

[15] Kissela B, Schneider A, Kleindorfer D, Khoury J, Miller R, Alwell K, et al. Stroke in a biracial population: The excess burden of stroke among blacks. Stroke. 2004;**35**(2):426-431

[16] Howard G, McCullough LD, Howard VJ. Stroke disparities. In: Stroke [Internet]. London, United Kingdom: Elsevier Ltd; 2022. pp. 179-186.e3. Available from: https://linkinghub.elsevier.com/retrieve/pii/B9780323694247000156

[17] Austin PC, Steyerberg EW. Events per variable (EPV) and the relative performance of different strategies for estimating the out-of-sample validity of logistic regression models. Statistical Methods in Medical Research. 2017;**26**(2):796-808

[18] Amarenco P, Abboud H, Labreuche J, Arauz A, Bryer A, Lavados PM, et al. Impact of living and socioeconomic characteristics on cardiovascular risk in ischemic stroke patients. International Journal of Stroke. 2014;**9**(8):1065-1072

[19] Cheng YC, Cole JW, Kittner SJ, Mitchell BD. Genetics of ischemic stroke in young adults. Circulation. Cardiovascular Genetics. 2014;**7**(3):383-392

[20] Terni E, Giannini N, Brondi M, Montano V, Bonuccelli U, Mancuso M. Genetics of ischaemic stroke in young adults. BBA Clinical. 2015;**3**:96-106

[21] He H, Pan Z, Wu J, Hu C, Bai L, Lyu J. Health effects of tobacco at the global, regional, and national levels: Results from the 2019 global burden of disease study. Nicotine & Tobacco Research: Official Journal of the Society for Research on Nicotine and Tobacco. 2022;**24**(6):864-870

[22] Lin F, Chen X, Shi Y, Yang K, Hu G, Zhuang W, et al. Early-life tobacco smoke exposure and stroke risk: A prospective study of 341,783 and 352,737 UK biobank participants. BMC Public Health. 2024;**24**(1):1339

[23] Pan B, Jin X, Jun L, Qiu S, Zheng Q, Pan M. The relationship between smoking and stroke: A meta-analysis. Medicine (Baltimore). 2019;**98**(12):e14872

[24] Salahuddin S, Prabhakaran D, Roy A. Pathophysiological mechanisms of tobacco-related CVD. Global Heart. 2012;**7**(2):113-120

[25] Owens AP, Mackman N. Tissue factor and thrombosis: The clot starts here. Thrombosis and Haemostasis. 2010;**104**(3):432-439

[26] Chung JW, Lee SR, Choi EK, Park SH, Lee H, Choi J, et al. Cumulative alcohol consumption burden and the risk of stroke in young adults: A nationwide population-based study. Neurology. 2023;**100**(5):e505-e515

[27] Hillbom M, Saloheimo P, Juvela S. Alcohol consumption, blood pressure, and the risk of stroke. Current Hypertension Reports. 2011;**13**(3):208-213

[28] Pietiläinen KH, Kaprio J, Borg P, Plasqui G, Yki-Järvinen H, Kujala UM, et al. Physical inactivity and obesity: A vicious circle. Obesity (Silver Spring, Md.). 2008;**16**(2):409-414

[29] Kohl HW, Craig CL, Lambert EV, Inoue S, Alkandari JR, Leetongin G, et al. The pandemic of physical inactivity: Global action for public health. The Lancet. 2012;**380**(9838):294-305

[30] Esse K, Fossati-Bellani M, Traylor A, Martin-Schild S. Epidemic of illicit drug

use, mechanisms of action/addiction and stroke as a health hazard. Brain and Behavior: A Cognitive Neuroscience Perspective. 2011;**1**(1):44-54

[31] Fonseca AC, Ferro JM. Drug abuse and stroke. Current Neurology and Neuroscience Reports. 2013;**13**(2):325

[32] Lappin JM, Darke S, Farrell M. Stroke and methamphetamine use in young adults: A review. Journal of Neurology, Neurosurgery, and Psychiatry. 2017;**88**(12):1079-1091

[33] Hagan IG, Burney K. Radiology of recreational drug abuse. Radiographics. 2007;**27**(4):919-940

[34] Johansson BB. Hypertension mechanisms causing stroke. Clinical and Experimental Pharmacology & Physiology. 1999;**26**(7):563-565

[35] Aiyagari V, Gorelick PB, editors. Hypertension and Stroke: Pathophysiology and Management. Cham: Springer International Publishing; 2016. Available from: http://link.springer.com/10.1007/978-3-319-29152-9

[36] Tun NN, Arunagirinathan G, Munshi SK, Pappachan JM. Diabetes mellitus and stroke: A clinical update. World Journal of Diabetes. 2017;**8**(6):235-248

[37] Poznyak A, Grechko AV, Poggio P, Myasoedova VA, Alfieri V, Orekhov AN. The diabetes mellitus–atherosclerosis connection: The role of lipid and glucose metabolism and chronic inflammation. International Journal of Molecular Sciences. 2020;**21**(5):1835

[38] Chen R, Ovbiagele B, Feng W. Diabetes and stroke: Epidemiology, pathophysiology, pharmaceuticals and outcomes. The American Journal of the Medical Sciences. 2016;**351**(4):380-386

[39] Ayata C, Shin HK, Dileköz E, Atochin DN, Kashiwagi S, Eikermann-Haerter K, et al. Hyperlipidemia disrupts cerebrovascular reflexes and worsens ischemic perfusion defect. Journal of Cerebral Blood Flow and Metabolism. 2013;**33**(6):954-962

[40] Xing Y, An Z, Yu N, Zhao W, Ning X, Wang J. Low density lipoprotein cholesterol and the outcome of acute ischemic stroke: Results of a large hospital-based study. European Neurology. 2016;**76**(5-6):195-201

[41] Ha SH, Kim BJ. Dyslipidemia treatment and cerebrovascular disease: Evidence regarding the mechanism of stroke. Journal of Lipid and Atherosclerosis. 2024;**13**(2):139

[42] Savelieva I, Bajpai A, John Camm A. Stroke in atrial fibrillation: Update on pathophysiology, new antithrombotic therapies, and evolution of procedures and devices. Annals of Medicine. 2007;**39**(5):371-391

[43] Sage JI, Van Uitert RL. Risk of recurrent stroke in patients with atrial fibrillation and non-valvular heart disease. Stroke. 1983;**14**(4):537-540

[44] Lin TT, Sung YL, Ko TY, Lee CK, Lin LY, Juang JJM, et al. Risk of ischemic stroke in patients with hypertrophic cardiomyopathy in the absence of atrial fibrillation—A nationwide cohort study. Aging. 2019;**11**(23):11347-11357

[45] Lanz J, Brophy JM, Therrien J, Kaouache M, Guo L, Marelli AJ. Stroke in adults with congenital heart disease: Incidence, cumulative risk, and predictors. Circulation. 2015;**132**(25):2385-2394

[46] Maheshwari R, Wardman D, Cordato DJ, Bhaskar SMM. Acute ischaemic stroke in infective

endocarditis: Pathophysiology and clinical outcomes in patients treated with reperfusion therapy. Immuno. 2021;**1**(4):347-359

[47] Mishra V, Banerjee A, Gandhi AB, Kaleem I, Alexander J, Hisbulla M, et al. Stroke and fabry disease: A review of literature. Cureus. 2020;**12**(12):e12083

[48] Chaughtai S, Chaughtai Z, Haider MS, Ijaz HM, Elmedani S, Bakr M, et al. Subacute stroke in a young female: A case of moyamoya syndrome initially anchoring with anxiety. Case Reports in Medicine. 2019;**2019**:7919568

[49] Murakami H, Ono K. MELAS: Mitochondrial encephalomyopathy, lactic acidosis and stroke-like episodes. Brain and Nerve = Shinkei Kenky No Shinpo. 2017;**69**(2):111-117

[50] Yang F, Peng S, Peng Q. Diagnosis of adult-onset MELAS with suspected recurrent strokes: A case report. Experimental and Therapeutic Medicine. 2022;**24**(1):466

[51] Harriott AM, Zimmerman E, Singhal AB, Jaff MR, Lindsay ME, Rordorf GA. Cerebrovascular fibromuscular dysplasia: The MGH cohort and literature review. Neurology Clinical Practice. 2017;7(3):225-236

[52] Topcuoglu MA, Singhal AB. Hemorrhagic reversible cerebral vasoconstriction syndrome: Features and mechanisms. Stroke. 2016;**47**(7):1742-1747

[53] Patel ML, Sachan R, Seth G. Combined deficiency of proteins C and S: Ischaemic stroke in young individuals. BML Case Reports. 2013;**2013**:bcr2012008016

[54] Graham JA, Daly HM, Carson PJ. Antithrombin III deficiency and cerebrovascular accidents in young adults. Journal of Clinical Pathology. 1992;**45**(10):921-922

[55] Hamedani AG, Cole JW, Mitchell BD, Kittner SJ. Meta-analysis of factor V Leiden and ischemic stroke in young adults: The importance of case ascertainment. Stroke. 2010;**41**(8):1599-1603

[56] Jiang B, Ryan KA, Hamedani A, Cheng Y, Sparks MJ, Koontz D, et al. Prothrombin G20210A mutation is associated with young-onset stroke: The genetics of early-onset stroke study and meta-analysis. Stroke. 2014;**45**(4):961-967

[57] Wiseman SJ, Bastin ME, Jardine CL, Barclay G, Hamilton IF, Sandeman E, et al. Cerebral small vessel disease burden is increased in systemic lupus erythematosus. Stroke. 2016;**47**(11):2722-2728

[58] Jordan LC, Casella JF, DeBaun MR. Prospects for primary stroke prevention in children with sickle cell anaemia. British Journal of Haematology. 2012;**157**(1):14-25

[59] Födinger M, Hörl WH, Sunder-Plassmann G. Molecular biology of 5,10-methylenetetrahydrofolate reductase. Journal of Nephrology. 2000;**13**(1):20-33

[60] Nedeltchev K. Ischaemic stroke in young adults: Predictors of outcome and recurrence. Journal of Neurology, Neurosurgery, and Psychiatry. 2005;**76**(2):191-195

[61] Debette S, Leys D. Cervical-artery dissections: Predisposing factors, diagnosis, and outcome. Lancet Neurology. 2009;**8**(7):668-678

[62] Ali Ebrahimi H, Hamzeaie Moghadam A, Aredestani E. Evaluation

of patent foramen ovale in young adults with cryptogenic stroke. ARYA Atherosclerosis. 2011;7(2):74-77

[63] Albers GW, Lansberg MG, Kemp S, Tsai JP, Lavori P, Christensen S, et al. A multicenter randomized controlled trial of endovascular therapy following imaging evaluation for ischemic stroke (DEFUSE 3). International Journal of Stroke: Official Journal of the International Stroke Society. 2017;**12**(8):896-905

[64] Greenberg SM, Ziai WC, Cordonnier C, Dowlatshahi D, Francis B, Goldstein JN, et al. 2022 guideline for the management of patients with spontaneous intracerebral hemorrhage: A guideline from the American Heart Association/American Stroke Association. Stroke. 2022;**53**(7):e282-e361

[65] Ojaghihaghighi S, Vahdati SS, Mikaeilpour A, Ramouz A. Comparison of neurological clinical manifestation in patients with hemorrhagic and ischemic stroke. World Journal of Emergency Medicine. 2017;**8**(1):34-38

[66] Hemphill JC, Greenberg SM, Anderson CS, Becker K, Bendok BR, Cushman M, et al. Guidelines for the management of spontaneous intracerebral hemorrhage: A guideline for healthcare professionals from the American Heart Association/American Stroke Association. Stroke. 2015;**46**(7):2032-2060

[67] Smajlović D. Strokes in young adults: Epidemiology and prevention. Vascular Health and Risk Management. 2015;**11**:157-164

[68] Khariton Y, House JA, Comer L, Coggins TR, Magalski A, Skolnick DG, et al. Impact of transesophageal echocardiography on management in patients with suspected cardioembolic stroke. The American Journal of Cardiology. 2014;**114**(12):1912-1916

[69] Mas JL, Derumeaux G, Guillon B, Massardier E, Hosseini H, Mechtouff L, et al. Patent foramen ovale closure or anticoagulation vs. antiplatelets after stroke. The New England Journal of Medicine. 2017;**377**(11):1011-1021

[70] Søndergaard L, Kasner SE, Rhodes JF, Andersen G, Iversen HK, Nielsen-Kudsk JE, et al. Patent foramen ovale closure or antiplatelet therapy for cryptogenic stroke. The New England Journal of Medicine. 2017;**377**(11):1033-1042

[71] Saver JL, Carroll JD, Thaler DE, Smalling RW, MacDonald LA, Marks DS, et al. Long-term outcomes of patent foramen ovale closure or medical therapy after stroke. The New England Journal of Medicine. 2017;**377**(11):1022-1032

[72] Sundell L, Salomaa V, Vartiainen E, Poikolainen K, Laatikainen T. Increased stroke risk is related to a binge-drinking habit. Stroke. 2008;**39**(12):3179-3184

[73] Dennis MS. Effective prophylaxis for deep vein thrombosis after stroke: Low-dose anticoagulation rather than stockings alone: Against. Stroke. 2004;**35**(12):2912-2913

[74] Winstein CJ, Stein J, Arena R, Bates B, Cherney LR, Cramer SC, et al. Guidelines for adult stroke rehabilitation and recovery: A guideline for healthcare professionals from the American Heart Association/American Stroke Association. Stroke. 2016;**47**(6):e98-e169

[75] Trapl M, Enderle P, Nowotny M, Teuschl Y, Matz K, Dachenhausen A, et al. Dysphagia bedside screening for acute-stroke patients: The Gugging swallowing screen. Stroke. 2007;**38**(11):2948-2952

[76] Stack CA, Cole JW. The clinical approach to stroke in young adults. In: Dehkharghani S, editor. Stroke. Brisbane, Australia: Exon Publications; 2021. pp. 53-78. Available from: https://exonpublications.com/index.php/exon/article/view/319

[77] Tabaac B, Dickstein L, Gurnea K, Hillis AE. Follow-up imaging after thrombolysis: FIAT, a randomized trial. Journal of Stroke and Cerebrovascular Diseases. 2023;**32**(6):107092

[78] Johnston SC, Easton JD, Farrant M, Barsan W, Conwit RA, Elm JJ, et al. Clopidogrel and aspirin in acute ischemic stroke and high-risk TIA. The New England Journal of Medicine. 2018;**379**(3):215-225

[79] Dong J, Wang F, Sundararajan S. Use of dual antiplatelet therapy following ischemic stroke. Stroke. 2020;**51**(5):e78-e80

[80] Saposnik G, Barinagar rementeria F, Brown RD, Bushnell CD, Cucchiara B, Cushman M, et al. Diagnosis and management of cerebral venous thrombosis: A statement for healthcare professionals from the American Heart Association/ American Stroke Association. Stroke. 2011;**42**(4):1158-1192

[81] Gaciong Z, Siński M, Lewandowski J. Blood pressure control and primary prevention of stroke: Summary of the recent clinical trial data and meta-analyses. Current Hypertension Reports. 2013;**15**(6):559-574

[82] Oesterle A, Laufs U, Liao JK. Pleiotropic effects of statins on the cardiovascular system. Circulation Research. 2017;**120**(1):229-243

[83] Castilla-Guerra L, Fernandez-Moreno MDC, Leon-Jimenez D, Carmona-Nimo E. Antidiabetic drugs and stroke risk. Current evidence. European Journal of Internal Medicine. 2018;**48**:1-5

[84] Teasell R, Foley N, Salter K, Bhogal S, Jutai J, Speechley M. Evidence-based review of stroke rehabilitation: Executive summary, 12th edition. Topics in Stroke Rehabilitation. 2009;**16**(6):463-488

Chapter 6

Carotid Stenosis as Stroke Risk Factor

Changyang Zhong, Jingxin Zhang, Cong Wu, Yinquan Sun, Wei Zhu, Yong Lu, Huiming Dou, Guochu Peng and Zhang Zuyong

Abstract

The study's comprehensive analysis of carotid stenosis and its mechanisms highlights the critical role of atherosclerotic plaques in stroke development. By integrating detailed pathophysiological insights with the latest diagnostic and therapeutic approaches, the chapter provides valuable evidence-based guidelines for clinicians. The review underscores the necessity of a multidisciplinary approach in managing carotid stenosis and ischemic stroke. Through a detailed exploration of risk factors, diagnostic techniques, and treatment strategies, the study not only enhances our understanding of the disease but also offers actionable recommendations to improve patient outcomes. The evidence presented is intended to influence both clinical practice and future research, ultimately contributing to the reduction of the global stroke burden. In conclusion, this chapter is a valuable resource for healthcare professionals, offering a detailed examination of carotid stenosis and its implications for ischemic stroke. By synthesizing current research with clinical practices, the study provides a robust foundation for optimizing stroke prevention and management strategies. Continued research and collaboration are essential to advancing our understanding and improving the quality of life for individuals affected by this pervasive health issue.

Keywords: carotid artery stenosis, ischemic stroke, atherosclerosis, plaque rupture, thromboembolism, carotid endarterectomy, stenting, medical therapy, asymptomatic stenosis, intrastent restenosis

1. Introduction

Stroke, characterized by acute focal neurological deficits, encompasses a spectrum of clinical syndromes, including hemiparesis, dysarthria, sensory loss, aphasia, and visual field deficits. Globally, stroke ranks as the second leading cause of death, claiming approximately 6 million lives annually [1]. While the age-standardized incidence of stroke has shown a declining trend, the absolute number of cases continues to rise due to population growth and aging. Of all stroke types, ischemic stroke constitutes approximately 70–80% of cases, establishing it as the most prevalent and clinically significant form [2].

A critical and independent risk factor for ischemic stroke is carotid artery stenosis, with an estimated 15% of first-time cerebrovascular events attributable to asymptomatic carotid artery stenosis leading to arterial thromboembolism [3]. Epidemiological studies across diverse global populations reveal that the prevalence of carotid artery atherosclerotic plaques among individuals aged 30 to 79 years is approximately 21.1%, affecting an estimated 815.76 million people. Among these, the prevalence of significant carotid artery stenosis is about 1.5%, impacting around 57.79 million individuals [4]. Given the global trend of population aging, the prevalence of carotid artery stenosis is poised to increase, thereby imposing a substantial burden on healthcare systems worldwide.

Carotid artery stenosis is defined as the narrowing of the carotid artery lumen, with atherosclerotic plaque formation representing the most prevalent etiological factor, accounting for approximately 90% of cases. Other causes include giant cell arteritis, fibromuscular dysplasia, arteritis, arterial tortuosity, trauma, tumors, and congenital arterial obliteration [5]. Atherosclerosis, a systemic disease characterized by the accumulation of lipid-rich plaques within arterial walls, represents a critical pathological substrate for carotid artery stenosis. The disease progression begins with intimal-medial thickening, followed by the formation of atherosclerotic plaques, which may eventually lead to lumen narrowing or occlusion [6]. This pathological process significantly escalates the risk of ischemic cerebrovascular events, including transient episodes of amaurosis fugax, transient ischemic attacks (TIAs), and ischemic stroke [7].

Given the profound implications of carotid artery stenosis for cerebrovascular morbidity and mortality, a standardized approach to its prevention and management is of paramount importance. This comprehensive review aims to systematically explore the pathophysiological mechanisms, risk factors, classification, diagnostic methodologies, and treatment strategies associated with carotid artery stenosis. Furthermore, the chapter provides an in-depth narrative on the current state of research and therapeutic advancements in the field. Through this systematic examination, the study seeks to enhance clinical understanding, inform evidence-based decision-making, and guide the development of targeted interventions to mitigate the adverse effects of carotid artery stenosis.

By synthesizing insights from contemporary research and established clinical practices, this review not only delineates the current knowledge but also highlights potential directions for future investigations. The ultimate goal is to contribute to a reduction in the global burden of cerebrovascular diseases through improved preventive and therapeutic strategies. This work serves as a valuable resource for clinicians, researchers, and healthcare providers engaged in the management of carotid artery stenosis and related cerebrovascular conditions, thereby advancing the field of neurovascular medicine.

1.1 Mechanisms of carotid stenosis leading to cerebral infarction

Carotid stenosis, predominantly caused by atherosclerosis (accounting for over 90% of cases), represents a significant contributor to the pathogenesis of ischemic stroke [8]. Atherosclerosis preferentially occurs at vascular bifurcations and regions where blood flow dynamics change direction or velocity, such as the carotid bulb, where the common carotid artery (CCA) divides into the internal and external carotid arteries [9]. This anatomical predisposition renders these regions particularly susceptible to the development of atherosclerotic lesions.

Atherosclerotic plaques are composed of a lipid-rich core, covered by a fibrous cap, and are classified as either stable or unstable (vulnerable) based on their histopathological characteristics [10]. Stable plaques exhibit a thick fibrous cap with a relatively small lipid core, which reduce the likelihood of rupture but still progress to cause arterial narrowing [11]. In contrast, unstable plaques are characterized by a thin fibrous cap, a large lipid core, and significant leukocytic infiltration, rendering them prone to rupture and subsequent acute vascular complications [12].

The mechanisms by which carotid stenosis contributes to cerebral infarction are complex and multifaceted, involving a combination of hemodynamic, structural, and thromboembolic factors:

1. *Plaque rupture and embolization:* The progression of atherosclerosis in the carotid artery can lead to the rupture of unstable plaques. This rupture releases cholesterol crystals, calcific debris, or other constituents of the plaque into the bloodstream, forming emboli. These embolic particles can travel through the cerebral circulation, obstructing smaller intracranial vessels and precipitating ischemic infarction [13].

2. *Thrombus formation and embolization:* Following plaque rupture or erosion, the exposure of underlying collagenous or elastotic tissue triggers platelet aggregation and the formation of a fibrin-rich thrombus. This thrombus may grow, obstruct the carotid lumen, or detach and travel to the brain, resulting in embolic stroke. The process of thrombus formation and embolization is further influenced by hemodynamic factors, such as flow velocity and shear stress, which promote thrombus stability or fragmentation [14].

3. *Vascular structural integrity compromise:* Ruptured or eroded plaques can compromise the structural integrity of the arterial wall, leading to intimal tears, media calcification, or intimal-medial separation (dissection) [15]. These structural disruptions can result in intramural hematomas, further arterial narrowing, or the development of recirculation zones, all of which contribute to cerebral ischemia.

4. *Altered hemodynamics:* As atherosclerotic plaques enlarge, they progressively narrow the carotid lumen, distorting blood flow patterns. This hemodynamic alteration can lead to areas of low or turbulent flow, which predispose to secondary thrombus formation and stabilization. In cases of severe stenosis (typically >70% lumen reduction), cerebral hypoperfusion may occur, even in the absence of overt thrombotic or embolic events, due to reduced blood supply to critical brain regions [16].

5. *Acute thrombotic occlusion* The acute rupture of a vulnerable plaque can precipitate rapid thrombus formation, leading to complete occlusion of the extracranial carotid artery. This thrombotic occlusion results in immediate cessation of cerebral blood flow to the ipsilateral hemisphere, causing complete ischemic infarction [17].

1.2 Clinical and pathophysiological implications

Understanding these mechanisms is essential for developing effective strategies to prevent and manage carotid stenosis. Each mechanism highlights the importance of early detection through imaging modalities such as carotid duplex ultrasonography or CT angiography, aggressive risk factor modification (e.g., lipid-lowering therapy, and antihypertensive and antiplatelet medications), and timely intervention in high-risk patients. Targeting vulnerable plaques, optimizing hemodynamic conditions, and preventing thrombus formation remain critical goals in the clinical management of carotid stenosis to reduce the global burden of ischemic stroke.

2. Risk factors and prevention of carotid artery stenosis

Carotid artery stenosis, a significant contributor to ischemic cerebrovascular events, arises from the cumulative effect of various risk factors. These factors are predominantly linked to atherosclerosis, a systemic disease characterized by the buildup of lipid-rich plaques in arterial walls. The primary risk factors for carotid artery stenosis can be categorized into modifiable (lifestyle-related) and non-modifiable (inherent) factors, each playing a critical role in the development and progression of the condition.

2.1 Hypertension

Hypertension stands as the foremost risk factor for cerebrovascular diseases, including carotid artery stenosis. Chronic elevation of arterial pressure leads to vascular wall damage, promoting the development of atherosclerotic lesions. The increased mechanical stress on the arterial walls accelerates the formation of intimal-medial thickening and the development of atherosclerotic plaques [18]. Studies have consistently shown that effective management of hypertension through antihypertensive therapy can significantly reduce the risk of cerebrovascular complications, including stroke and transient ischemic attacks (TIAs) [19]. Optimal blood pressure control, typically targeting a systolic pressure below 130 mmHg and diastolic pressure below 80 mmHg, is essential for mitigating the vascular damage associated with hypertension [20].

2.2 Age

Advanced age is a primary non-modifiable risk factor for carotid artery stenosis, with incidence increasing steadily from middle age onwards. The condition is particularly prevalent among individuals aged 60 years and older, reflecting the cumulative effects of vascular aging and atherosclerotic progression. Age-related changes, such as reduced endothelial function and increased arterial stiffness, contribute to the development of atherosclerotic plaques [21]. While age itself cannot be modified, understanding its impact is crucial for targeted screening and preventive interventions in older populations.

2.3 Smoking

Cigarette smoking emerges as a major modifiable contributor to carotid artery stenosis, with studies indicating a more than 50% increased risk among smokers compared to non-smokers. Smoking induces oxidative stress, leading to endothelial dysfunction and accelerated atherosclerosis. The toxic substances in cigarette smoke, such as nicotine, carbon monoxide, and free radicals, impair vascular endothelial cell function, promote inflammation, and enhance platelet aggregation. Quit smoking remains a critical component of preventive strategies, as it can significantly reduce the risk of developing carotid artery stenosis and related cerebrovascular events. Nicotine replacement therapy and behavioral interventions are effective aids for smoking cessation [22].

2.4 Diabetes mellitus

Diabetes mellitus contributes significantly to vascular inflammation and endothelial dysfunction, both of which promote the formation and progression of atherosclerotic plaques in the carotid arteries. Elevated blood glucose levels in diabetic patients lead to increased glycation of LDL-C, rendering it more oxidized and atherogenic [23]. Additionally, diabetes is associated with metabolic abnormalities, including insulin resistance and dyslipidemia, which further predispose individuals to atherosclerosis. Glycemic control, achieved through a combination of lifestyle modifications and pharmacological agents, is essential in mitigating these effects and reducing the risk of cerebrovascular complications.

2.5 Hyperlipidemia

Elevated levels of low-density lipoprotein cholesterol (LDL-C) are directly associated with the development of atherosclerotic plaques. LDL-C transports cholesterol to the arterial wall, where it can become oxidized and retained, leading to plaque formation [24]. Conversely, high levels of high-density lipoprotein cholesterol (HDL-C) are protective, as HDL facilitates the removal of excess cholesterol from the arterial wall. Statin therapy has been conclusively demonstrated to reduce stroke risk by lowering LDL-C levels and slowing the progression of intimal-medial thickening in the carotid arteries. Current guidelines emphasize stratified LDL-C targets for primary and secondary prevention. The 2023 ACC/AHA Clinical Guideline Update recommends maintaining LDL-C < 70 mg/dL (1.8 mmol/L) for very high-risk populations (e.g., established ASCVD or diabetes with multiple risk factors), and < 100 mg/dL (2.6 mmol/L) for moderate-risk individuals [25].

2.6 Other risk factors

Additional modifiable risk factors include obesity, sedentary lifestyle, and poor dietary habits. Obesity, particularly abdominal obesity, is associated with metabolic syndrome, which encompasses hyperlipidemia, hypertension, and insulin resistance—conditions that collectively increase the risk of atherosclerosis [26]. A sedentary lifestyle is linked to reduced high-density lipoprotein (HDL) levels and increased LDL levels, both of which favor plaque formation. Poor dietary habits, characterized by high intake of saturated fats, trans fats, salt, and sugar, contribute to dyslipidemia and hypertension, thereby increasing the risk of carotid artery stenosis [27].

Non-modifiable risk factors encompass cardiovascular disease family history and elevated levels of C-reactive protein (CRP), a marker of systemic inflammation. A family history of cardiovascular diseases suggests a genetic predisposition to atherosclerosis, highlighting the importance of heightened vigilance and early intervention in such individuals. Elevated CRP levels indicate an underlying inflammatory state, which accelerates atherosclerotic progression and increases the risk of vascular events [28].

2.7 Prevention strategies

The prevention of carotid artery stenosis involves a comprehensive, multi-pronged approach that addresses both modifiable and non-modifiable risk factors. Lifestyle modifications are foundational to risk reduction and include:

- *Adopting a healthy diet*: A diet rich in fruits, vegetables, whole grains, and foods high in omega-3 fatty acids (e.g., fatty fish, nuts, and seeds) can help reduce the risk of atherosclerosis. Limiting the intake of saturated fats, trans fats, salt, and sugar is crucial for maintaining optimal lipid and blood pressure levels [29].

- *Engaging in regular physical activity*: A minimum of 150 minutes of moderate-intensity aerobic exercise per week, such as brisk walking, cycling, or swimming, is recommended to promote cardiovascular health. Resistance training and flexibility exercises should also be included to improve overall fitness and reduce metabolic syndrome-related risks [30].

- *Avoiding tobacco and limiting alcohol consumption*: Smoking cessation is essential, and alcohol consumption should be limited to no more than one drink per day for women and two for men to minimize its impact on blood pressure and cholesterol levels [31].

Pharmacological interventions are integral to managing underlying conditions and reducing risk:

- *Statins for hyperlipidemia*: Statins are the cornerstone of lipid management, significantly reducing LDL-C levels and slowing atherosclerotic progression. They also provide additional benefits by reducing inflammation and oxidative stress.

- *Antihypertensives for blood pressure control*: Medications such as angiotensin-converting enzyme (ACE) inhibitors, ARBs, thiazide diuretics, and calcium channel blockers are effective in controlling hypertension. These agents not only reduce blood pressure but also possess additional vascular protective effects [32].

- *Antidiabetics for glycemic control*: Pharmacological agents such as metformin, sulfonylureas, and GLP-1 receptor agonists help achieve glycemic control, reducing the risk of atherosclerosis-related complications [33].

Regular medical screening is essential, particularly for individuals at high risk. Screening modalities such as carotid duplex ultrasonography and magnetic resonance imaging (MRI) can detect early signs of carotid artery stenosis and guide timely intervention. Periodic assessment of risk factors, including blood pressure, lipid profiles, and fasting glucose levels, allows for early identification of individuals at risk and timely implementation of preventive measures.

Understanding and addressing both modifiable and non-modifiable risk factors are essential for minimizing the incidence of carotid artery stenosis and its attendant cerebrovascular complications. A holistic approach that combines lifestyle modifications, pharmacological interventions, and regular medical monitoring is crucial for effective prevention and management. By reducing the burden of carotid artery stenosis, such strategies contribute to a significant reduction in the global prevalence of ischemic stroke and improve overall cardiovascular health.

3. Grading of the severity of carotid artery stenosis

The grading of carotid artery stenosis is primarily based on the degree of arterial lumen narrowing, as defined by large-scale clinical trials such as the North American Symptomatic Carotid Endarterectomy Trial (NASCET) and the European Carotid Surgery Trial (ECST) [34]. These studies have established a classification system that correlates the extent of stenosis with its clinical implications and treatment strategies. Below is a detailed grading system based on the percentage of arterial narrowing (**Figure 1**).

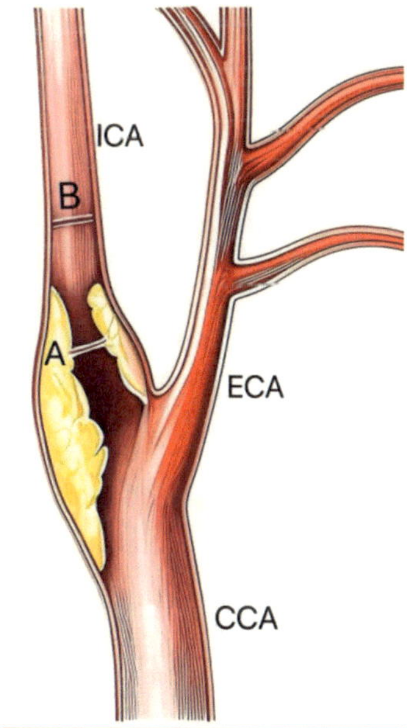

Figure 1.
Calculation of ICA stenosis according to the NASCET method. According to the NASCET study design, percent ICA stenosis is calculated by comparing the diameter of the residual lumen (A) to the diameter of the distal normal ICA (B). According to the ECST method for calculating ICA stenosis. Based on the ECST study design, the percentage of ICA stenosis is calculated by comparing the residual lumen diameter with the ICA lumen diameter at the stenotic site.

3.1 Mild stenosis: Stenosis <30%

Mild carotid artery stenosis, defined as a narrowing of less than 30% of the arterial lumen, typically exhibits minimal hemodynamic significance. At this stage, the flow reserve is preserved, and the risk of ischemic events is relatively low. Patients with mild stenosis generally do not require surgical or interventional treatment, but periodic monitoring is recommended to assess disease progression. Management at this stage primarily focuses on risk factor modification, such as lipid-lowering therapy, blood pressure control, and smoking cessation, to prevent disease progression. Regular imaging surveillance, such as carotid duplex ultrasonography, is essential to detect any progression of stenosis and to guide future management decisions.

3.2 Moderate stenosis: 30–70%

Moderate stenosis, characterized by a narrowing ranging from 30 to 70%, may lead to subtle hemodynamic changes. While the lumen is still sufficiently patent to maintain adequate blood flow under normal conditions, the vessel may become vulnerable to ischemic events during periods of increased demand, such as exercise or stress. The clinical significance at this stage is variable, and treatment decisions are often based on the presence of symptoms, such as transient ischemic attacks (TIAs) or minor strokes, as well as the overall cardiovascular risk profile of the patient. Asymptomatic individuals with moderate stenosis may be managed conservatively with intensive medical therapy, including statins, antihypertensives, and antiplatelet agents, to reduce the risk of progression and vascular events. However, patients with symptoms or high-risk features, such as advanced age, diabetes mellitus, or evidence of high-risk plaque, may be candidates for revascularization procedures [35].

3.3 Severe stenosis: 70–99%

Severe carotid artery stenosis, defined as a narrowing of 70 to 99%, is associated with a significantly increased risk of ischemic stroke due to the high likelihood of plaque rupture, thrombus formation, or embolic events. The hemodynamic reserve is significantly compromised, and even minor changes in blood flow dynamics can lead to critical reductions in cerebral perfusion, particularly during activities that increase cerebral metabolic demand. According to clinical guidelines, patients with severe stenosis, particularly those with symptoms, are strong candidates for revascularization procedures, such as carotid endarterectomy or carotid artery stenting, to reduce the risk of stroke. However, the decision to proceed with surgery or stenting is influenced by individual patient factors, such as age, comorbidities, and the presence of protective collateral circulation. Surgical intervention is generally recommended for symptomatic patients with severe stenosis, as it significantly reduces the risk of stroke compared to medical therapy alone. Additionally, the presence of high-risk plaque features, such as intraplaque hemorrhage, calcification, or a thick fibrous cap, further underscores the urgency for revascularization [36].

3.4 Complete occlusion: 100% stenosis

Complete occlusion of the carotid artery represents the most severe form of stenosis, where the lumen is entirely blocked by atherosclerotic plaque or a thrombus.

In this case, blood flow through the affected vessel is entirely absent, necessitating reliance on collateral circulation from the contralateral vertebral artery to maintain cerebral perfusion. Complete occlusion is associated with a high risk of ischemic stroke, particularly in the absence of adequate collateral flow. Patients with complete occlusion often present with recurrent TIAs or strokes, highlighting the urgency for intervention. The management of complete occlusion typically involves a comprehensive evaluation of collateral circulation, often through imaging modalities such as CT angiography or MR angiography [37]. Revascularization options, including carotid endarterectomy, stenting, or thrombectomy, are considered on a case-by-case basis, depending on the feasibility of restoring blood flow and the patient's overall clinical status.

3.5 Clinical implications and management strategies

The classification of carotid artery stenosis into these distinct grades provides a framework for clinical decision-making. It allows healthcare providers to tailor treatment plans based on the severity of stenosis and the associated risk of ischemic events. While mild and moderate stenosis are primarily managed through risk factor modification and medical therapy, severe and complete stenosis often require invasive interventions to mitigate the high risk of stroke.

Prompt and accurate diagnosis of carotid artery stenosis is critical, as delays in treatment can lead to devastating neurological complications. The integration of imaging modalities, such as carotid duplex ultrasonography, CT angiography, and magnetic resonance angiography (MRA), plays a pivotal role in the precise grading of stenosis and the detection of high-risk plaque features, such as intraplaque hemorrhage or calcification. Advanced imaging techniques, such as virtual histology or intravascular ultrasound, may also be employed to assess the composition of the atherosclerotic plaque, further guiding clinical decision-making [38].

In conclusion, the grading system for carotid artery stenosis, as outlined by the NASCET and ECST criteria, serves as a cornerstone for the management of patients with cerebrovascular disease. By correlating the degree of stenosis with its clinical significance, clinicians can optimize treatment strategies to improve patient outcomes and reduce the burden of ischemic stroke. The integration of clinical, hemodynamic, and imaging data is essential for accurately grading stenosis and implementing personalized treatment plans that address the unique needs of each patient.

4. Diagnosis of carotid artery stenosis

The diagnosis of carotid artery stenosis requires a comprehensive approach that integrates clinical symptoms, physical examination findings, and advanced imaging modalities. This section outlines the detailed process for diagnosing carotid artery stenosis, emphasizing both symptomatic and asymptomatic presentations, as well as the role of various diagnostic techniques.

4.1 Clinical presentation

Carotid artery stenosis can be categorized into two main clinical presentations: symptomatic and asymptomatic.

4.1.1 Asymptomatic carotid artery stenosis

Asymptomatic carotid artery stenosis refers to cases where patients exhibit no symptoms of ischemic brain injury, such as transient ischemic attacks (TIAs) or strokes, for at least 6 months prior to diagnosis. These individuals are often identified during routine health screenings or through imaging studies conducted for unrelated reasons, while symptom-free, asymptomatic patients may still harbor significant stenosis that could predispose them to future cerebrovascular events. Therefore, diagnostic evaluation remains crucial, particularly in high-risk populations such as those with a family history of cardiovascular disease, hypertension, diabetes mellitus, or other atherosclerotic risk factors.

4.1.2 Symptomatic carotid artery stenosis

Symptomatic carotid artery stenosis is defined by the presence of ischemic stroke or transient ischemic attack (TIA) within the past 6 months. The clinical manifestations are diverse and depend on the extent of stenosis and the specific areas of the brain affected.

4.1.2.1 Transient ischemic attack (TIA)

TIA represents a reversible neurological deficit caused by focal cerebral ischemia. Common symptoms include [39]:

- *Monocular blindness (amaurosis fugax)*: A sudden, transient loss of vision in one eye, often lasting minutes to hours due to thromboembolic occlusion of the ophthalmic artery.
- *Hemiparesis or hemisensory disturbance*: Acute onset of weakness or numbness on one side of the body, resulting from decreased blood flow to the brain's motor or sensory cortex.
- *Dysphasia or aphasia*: Difficulty with speech or language comprehension, indicative of involvement of the language centers in the brain.
- *Ataxia or vertigo*: Impaired coordination or a sense of dizziness, often caused by cerebellar ischemia.

TIA symptoms typically resolve within 24 hours without residual neurological deficits, as evidenced by normal neuroimaging studies.

4.1.2.2 Ischemic stroke

Ischemic stroke occurs when there is a sudden reduction or complete obstruction of blood flow to a portion of the brain, leading to tissue infarction and permanent neurological damage. Symptoms include [40]:

- *Hemiplegia or hemiparesis*: Complete or partial paralysis of one side of the body due to cortical or subcortical infarction.
- *Aphasia or dysarthria*: Impaired speech or difficulty forming words, reflecting damage to the language centers or motor pathways.

- *Sensory loss*: Loss of sensation or altered sensory perception, often corresponding to the brain region affected by the infarction.
- *Visual field deficits*: Loss of vision in specific areas of the visual field, resulting from infarction in the occipital lobe or its afferent pathways.
- *Cognitive impairment*: Confusion, memory loss, or executive dysfunction, particularly in cases of lacunar or watershed infarcts.

4.1.2.3 Other ischemic symptoms

Patients may also present with less common or nonspecific symptoms, such as:

- *Hemiphenomena*: A constellation of symptoms including ipsilateral Horner syndrome (ptosis, miosis, and anhidrosis) and contralateral hemisensory symptoms, often indicative of carotid artery dissection or severe stenosis.
- *Postural symptoms*: Dizziness or lightheadedness that worsens with changes in head position, possibly due to altered cerebral blood flow or orthostatic hypotension.
- *Cognitive dysfunction*: Transient or chronic deficits in attention, memory, or executive functioning, potentially resulting from multiple small vessel infarcts or chronic hypoperfusion.

These symptoms are often attributed to altered cerebral blood flow dynamics, such as hypoperfusion in the anterior or posterior circulation [41].

4.2 Physical examination

A thorough physical examination is essential to identify and characterize carotid artery stenosis. Key components include:

4.2.1 Carotid auscultation

Auscultation of the carotid arteries involves listening for vascular sounds, most commonly a bruit, which is a vascular noise typically heard during systole. A bruit suggests the presence of arterial narrowing or turbulence caused by atherosclerotic plaques [42]. However, the absence of a bruit does not exclude stenosis, as smaller plaques or those located in specific anatomical regions may not produce audible turbulence.

4.2.2 Ophthalmoscopic examination

Fundus examination may reveal ophthalmic manifestations of carotid artery stenosis [43], such as:

- *Sellar calcifications*: Calcifications in the sella turcica, often reflective of atherosclerotic plaques in the carotid arteries.
- *Hyaline plaques*: Yellowish, semi-transparent lesions in the retinal arteries, indicative of atherosclerosis.

4.2.3 Neurological examination

A detailed neurological assessment is crucial to identify and quantify any neurologic deficits. Key components include:

- *Motor examination*: Assessment of muscle strength, tone, and coordination to detect hemiparesis or ataxia.
- *Sensory examination*: Evaluation of sensation, including light touch, pain, and proprioception, to identify sensory loss.
- *Reflex evaluation*: Assessment of cranial nerves and deep tendon reflexes to detect abnormalities.
- *Cognitive assessment*: Testing of attention, memory, and language function to identify cognitive deficits.

4.3 Imaging modalities

Accurate diagnosis of carotid artery stenosis requires the use of advanced imaging techniques, particularly in symptomatic patients. The choice of imaging modality depends on the clinical context, patient comorbidities, and the availability of resources.

4.3.1 Carotid color-coded duplex sonography

Carotid duplex ultrasonography is the preferred initial imaging modality for screening and evaluating carotid artery stenosis [44]. This non-invasive technique combines B-mode imaging with pulsed-wave Doppler to provide:

- *Anatomical information*: High-resolution visualization of the arterial walls and lumen.
- *Hemodynamic data*: Measurement of peak systolic velocity and flow volume to estimate stenosis severity.
- *Plaque characterization*: Assessment of plaque composition based on echogenicity, with hypoechoic plaques indicative of lipid-rich, unstable plaques.

The advantages of ultrasound include its non-invasive nature, low cost, and wide availability. However, its accuracy is highly operator-dependent, and it may not provide imaging of the aortic arch or distal intracranial arteries. Additionally, ultrasound struggles to differentiate between mild, hemodynamically insignificant stenosis and moderate-to-severe narrowing.

4.3.2 Magnetic resonance angiography (MRA)

MRA is a non-invasive imaging modality that generates high-resolution images of the carotid arteries using magnetic resonance technology. Techniques such as 3D time-of-flight (TOF) imaging are employed to visualize the arterial lumen [45]. Key advantages of MRA include:

- *No ionizing radiation*: Safe for patients with contraindications to CT scanning.
- *No need for iodinated contrast*: Useful in patients with renal insufficiency.

Despite its advantages, MRA has several limitations:

- *Overestimation of stenosis*: MRA may exaggerate the degree of narrowing, particularly in cases of severe stenosis or occlusion.
- *Poor visualization of distal intracranial vessels*: MRA is less effective in imaging the distal cerebral circulation, limiting its utility in assessing intracranial aneurysms or vasospasm.

4.3.3 Computed tomography angiography (CTA)

CTA is a widely used imaging technique that provides detailed cross-sectional images of the carotid arteries [45]. It involves the intravenous administration of iodinated contrast medium, followed by high-resolution imaging using a CT scanner. CTA offers:

- *Detailed anatomical representation*: Clear depiction of the entire arterial tree, including the aortic arch, carotid bifurcation, and intracranial arteries.
- *Quantification of stenosis*: Accurate measurement of the ratio between the stenotic and normal vessel diameters.
- *Preoperative planning*: Useful for surgical planning in patients undergoing carotid endarterectomy.

The disadvantages of CTA include:

- *Radiation exposure*: Cumulative ionizing radiation is a concern, particularly for patients requiring repeated imaging.
- *Contrast nephropathy*: Risk of acute kidney injury in patients with pre-existing renal impairment.
- *Limited resolution*: CTA may fail to visualize small intracranial arteries or provide insufficient detail in cases of vascular tortuosity.

4.3.4 Digital subtraction angiography (DSA)

DSA is considered the gold standard for the diagnosis of carotid artery stenosis. This invasive technique involves the introduction of a catheter into the arterial system, followed by the injection of iodinated contrast medium. Digital imaging software is used to subtract background bone and soft tissue from the image, resulting in clear visualization of the arterial anatomy. DSA provides [46]:

- *High spatial resolution*: Accurate measurement of stenosis and identification of associated abnormalities such as aneurysms or vasospasm.
- *Therapeutic capabilities*: The ability to perform percutaneous interventions, such as carotid stenting, during the same procedure.

The drawbacks of DSA include:

- *Invasiveness*: Potential complications such as access site hematoma, infection, or catheter-induced arterial injury.

- *Cost and radiation*: Higher expense and exposure to ionizing radiation compared to non-invasive modalities.

- *Limited patient access*: Contraindications in patients with bleeding disorders, severe renal insufficiency, or allergies to contrast agents.

4.4 Diagnostic workflow

The diagnostic process for carotid artery stenosis begins with a thorough clinical evaluation, including a detailed history and physical examination. For symptomatic patients, imaging studies are essential to confirm the diagnosis and assess the extent of stenosis. The choice of imaging modality depends on clinical context, patient comorbidities, and the availability of advanced imaging techniques.

- *Initial screening*: Carotid duplex ultrasonography is often the first-line imaging modality due to its non-invasive nature, cost-effectiveness, and ability to provide both anatomical and hemodynamic information.

- *Definitive diagnosis*: For patients with significant stenosis or symptomatic disease, CTA or MRA is typically used to provide detailed anatomical information and confirm the diagnosis.

- *Preinterventional assessment*: DSA remains the standard for patients undergoing revascularization procedures, as it allows for both diagnostic and therapeutic interventions in a single procedure.

In conclusion, the accurate diagnosis of carotid artery stenosis requires a multifaceted approach that integrates clinical acumen with advanced imaging techniques. By carefully evaluating clinical symptoms, physical examination findings, and imaging data, healthcare providers can optimize patient outcomes and guide appropriate management strategies. The choice of diagnostic modality should be tailored to the individual patient's clinical profile and the need for accurate, timely diagnosis.

5. Surgical treatment

The clinical management of carotid artery stenosis involves both surgical intervention and conservative therapy. Surgical intervention is recommended for patients with high-risk stenosis who meet specific anatomic and clinical criteria. The two primary surgical procedures currently employed are carotid endarterectomy (CEA) and carotid artery stenting (CAS). The choice between these procedures is determined by a comprehensive evaluation of the patient's clinical condition, anatomic features, and adherence to evidence-based guidelines. The goal is to develop an individualized treatment plan that optimizes outcomes while minimizing complications [47].

5.1 Carotid endarterectomy (CEA)

CEA is the preferred treatment for patients with moderate-to-severe carotid artery stenosis, particularly in those with symptoms or unstable plaques. It is widely recognized as the gold standard for removing atherosclerotic plaques from the carotid arteries and is associated with long-term durable outcomes [48].

5.1.1 Indications

The indications for CEA are based on the severity of stenosis, clinical symptoms, and anatomic considerations. They are categorized into absolute and relative criteria.

Absolute indications

- *Symptomatic carotid artery stenosis*: Patients who have experienced a transient ischemic attack (TIA) or non-disabling stroke within the past 6 months attributed to carotid artery disease. CEA is strongly recommended to reduce the risk of recurrent cerebrovascular events.

- *Severe asymptomatic stenosis*: Patients without symptoms but with documented stenosis of 70% or greater in the internal carotid artery. Such high-grade stenosis confers a significant risk of future cerebrovascular events, even in asymptomatic patients.

5.2 Relative indications

- *Moderate asymptomatic stenosis*: Patients with 50–69% stenosis who are asymptomatic but at heightened risk for cerebrovascular events due to comorbidities such as age, diabetes mellitus, or hypertension.

- *Unstable plaques*: Patients with acute or subacute strokes, TIAs, or imaging evidence of high-risk plaque characteristics, such as calcified, hemorrhagic, or ulcerated plaques.

- *Bilateral carotid artery disease*: Patients with significant stenosis in both carotid arteries. In such cases, surgical intervention is often advised for both sides, prioritizing the symptomatic or more severely affected vessel.

5.2.1 Contraindications

While CEA is a well-established and effective procedure, it is not universally indicated. Contraindications include:

- *Chronic asymptomatic stenosis*: Patients with no clinical symptoms and stable, asymptomatic stenosis. In such cases, medical therapy and imaging surveillance may suffice.

- *Recent neurovascular events*: Patients who have experienced a stroke or intracranial hemorrhage within the past 3 months.

- *Recent myocardial infarction*: Patients who have had a myocardial infarction within the past 2 weeks.

- *Severe cognitive impairment*: Patients with advanced dementia or inability to provide informed consent.

- *Hematological disorders*: Patients with coagulation disorders or contraindications to anticoagulant therapy.
- *Severe comorbidities*: Patients with end-stage organ disease or conditions that render surgery inherently high-risk.

5.2.2 Preoperative preparation

Comprehensive preoperative preparation is critical to optimize surgical outcomes and minimize perioperative risks.

- *Medical optimization*: Patients should be maintained on antiplatelet therapy, typically aspirin or clopidogrel, starting at least 4 days prior to surgery. This reduces the risk of perioperative thromboembolic events.
- *Hypertension management*: Blood pressure should be controlled to a target range of <140/90 mmHg to reduce the risk of intraoperative complications.
- *Lipid regulation*: Statin therapy is continued perioperatively to stabilize plaques and reduce inflammation.
- *Cardiac assessment*: A thorough evaluation of cardiac function is conducted, including echocardiography and electrocardiographic monitoring, to ensure safe anesthesia and minimize cardiovascular risks.
- *Imaging studies*: Preoperative imaging, such as duplex ultrasound, CT angiography, or magnetic resonance angiography (MRA), is performed to confirm stenosis severity and guide surgical planning.

5.2.3 Surgical technique

The surgical procedure for CEA involves the following steps:

1. *Patient positioning*: The patient is placed in the supine position, with the head turned slightly away from the side of the lesion.
2. *Anesthesia*: General anesthesia is typically used to ensure patient comfort and immobility during the procedure.
3. *Skin incision*: A longitudinal incision is made along the anterior border of the sternocleidomastoid muscle, extending from the mastoid process to the supraclavicular region.
4. *Vascular exposure*: The cervical fascia is dissected to expose the carotid sheath. The common carotid artery, internal carotid artery, and external carotid artery are carefully mobilized, with attention to preserving nearby structures such as the vagus nerve and hypoglossal nerve.
5. *Arterial occlusion*: After achieving hemostasis with temporary clamping, the internal carotid artery is subjected to proximal and distal occlusion using vascular clamps or a carotid shunt to maintain cerebral perfusion.

6. *Plaque removal*: The internal carotid artery is transected, and the atherosclerotic plaque is excised. The intimal flap is carefully removed, ensuring smooth margins and complete eradication of the lesion.

7. *Vascular reconstruction*: The artery is repaired using sutures or a synthetic patch if necessary, restoring the arterial lumen to its normal caliber.

8. *Reperfusion*: The clamps are gradually removed, and the patency of the internal carotid artery is confirmed via palpation or Doppler ultrasound.

9. *Wound closure*: The incision is closed, and the patient is monitored in the recovery area for any signs of complications, such as hematoma or infection.

5.2.4 Postoperative care

Postoperative care is essential to ensure neurologic and cardiovascular stability and to minimize the risk of complications.

- *Antiplatelet therapy*: Patients are maintained on aspirin or another antiplatelet agent for at least 4 weeks to prevent thrombosis. Dual antiplatelet therapy may be prescribed for a short period postoperatively.

- *Neurological monitoring*: Patients are closely monitored for any signs of neurologic deficits, such as aphasia, hemiparesis, or sensory abnormalities.

- *Imaging surveillance*: A postoperative duplex ultrasound is performed to assess the patency of the artery and the integrity of the repair.

- *Medication management*: Continuation of statin therapy and blood pressure control is recommended to optimize long-term outcomes.

- *Lifestyle modification*: Patients are encouraged to adopt a heart-healthy lifestyle, including smoking cessation, dietary changes, and regular exercise, to reduce the risk of future cardiovascular events.

5.3 Carotid artery stenting (CAS)

CAS is an alternative treatment option for patients with severe carotid artery stenosis who are at high surgical risk or have anatomic factors that complicate endarterectomy. This minimally invasive procedure involves the placement of a stent within the narrowed artery to restore blood flow. CAS is particularly suitable for patients with high-risk anatomy, such as lesions involving the carotid bifurcation or patients with a history of cerebellar symptoms post-CEA [49].

5.3.1 Indications

CAS is considered for the following clinical scenarios:

- *Symptomatic carotid artery stenosis*: Patients with moderate-to-severe stenosis who are at elevated risk for surgery due to comorbidities or anatomic constraints.

- *Asymptomatic carotid artery stenosis*: Patients with 70–99% stenosis and no symptoms but at high risk for cerebrovascular events. However, the clinical utility of CAS in asymptomatic patients remains under investigation [50].

5.3.2 Contraindications

CAS is contraindicated in the following situations:

- *Extensive calcification*: Lesions involving long segments of the carotid artery that may preclude effective stent deployment.
- *Anatomic constraints*: Severe tortuosity of the aortic arch or other vascular anomalies that prevent adequate access or stent placement.
- *Contraindications to CEA*: These include patients with cerebellar ataxia, ipsilateral carotid artery myoclonus, or significant vocal cord palsy from previous CEA.

5.3.3 Preoperative preparation

Preoperative preparation for CAS is critical to ensure safety and efficacy.

- *Antiplatelet therapy*: Patients begin taking aspirin and clopidogrel at least 1 week before surgery. On the day of the procedure, a loading dose of clopidogrel (300–600 mg) is administered. Alternative antiplatelet agents, such as ticagrelor or prasugrel, may be used if the patient is intolerant to clopidogrel.
- *Blood pressure control*: Strict management of hypertension to a target range of <130/80 mmHg to reduce the risk of intraoperative complications.
- *Neurological assessment*: Continuous neurological evaluation is performed pre- and post-procedure, with the detailed documentation of neurological status for the first 24 hours.
- *Cardiac evaluation*: Assessment includes echocardiography and 24-hour Holter monitoring to evaluate cardiac function. Patients with bradycardia (heart rate < 50 bpm) or severe AV block may require temporary pacemaker placement during the procedure.
- *Peripheral vascular assessment*: Evaluation of peripheral artery integrity, including palpation of bilateral femoral and dorsalis pedis arteries, with additional imaging if necessary.
- *Lipid regulation*: Statin therapy is continued perioperatively to stabilize plaques and reduce inflammation [50].

5.3.4 Surgical technique

The procedure for CAS involves the following steps:

1. *Patient positioning*: The patient is placed in the supine position, with monitoring equipment connected. A small cushion is placed under the shoulder to slightly extend the neck, optimizing access to the femoral or radial artery.

2. *Skin preparation*: The surgical site is prepared and draped under sterile conditions. The femoral or radial artery is typically chosen as the access site.

3. *Vascular access*: Access is gained using the Seldinger technique, involving skin puncture, introducer sheath placement, and vessel dilation.

4. *Catheter placement and angiography*: Under fluoroscopic guidance, a guide wire is advanced to the target lesion. Selective angiography is performed to delineate the extent and severity of stenosis.

5. *Brain protection*: A distal protection device, such as an intracranial filter, is deployed to capture any embolic material released during the procedure.

6. *Pre-stent expansion*: A balloon dilation catheter is used to pre-stent the narrowed segment, ensuring adequate vessel preparation for stent deployment.

7. *Stent deployment*: The appropriately sized self-expanding or balloon-expandable stent is positioned at the lesion site and deployed to restore blood flow.

8. *Post-stent expansion and protection device retrieval*: If necessary, the stent is further expanded. After confirming satisfactory stent placement, the protection device is carefully retrieved.

9. *Procedure completion*: A final angiogram is performed to ensure patency of the artery. The catheter and sheath are withdrawn, and manual pressure is applied to the access site to achieve hemostasis. Alternatively, a vascular closure device may be used.

10. *Postoperative monitoring*: The patient is monitored in the recovery area, with particular attention to neurologic status, renal function (especially in patients with pre-existing renal impairment), and wound care at the access site.

5.3.5 Postoperative care

Following CAS, patients require vigilant postoperative monitoring and management.

- *Antiplatelet therapy*: Patients commence dual antiplatelet therapy immediately post-procedure, typically continuing for 1–3 months. This is followed by long-term maintenance therapy with aspirin or another antiplatelet agent.

- *Imaging follow-up*: Regular postoperative imaging, such as CT angiography or duplex ultrasound, is conducted to ensure stent patency and exclude complications like restenosis or thrombosis.

- *Medication management*: Continuation of statin therapy and blood pressure control is recommended to reduce the risk of restenosis and optimize long-term outcomes.

- *Lifestyle advice*: Patients are encouraged to adopt a heart-healthy lifestyle, including smoking cessation, a low-fat diet, and regular exercise, to reduce the risk of future cardiovascular events [51].

5.4 Selection of surgical approach

The choice between CEA and CAS requires a comprehensive evaluation of multiple factors, including the patient's overall health, anatomic features, and lesion characteristics. CEA is generally preferred for patients with straightforward anatomic lesions and low surgical risk. CAS is favored for high-risk patients, those with anatomic complexities unsuitable for surgery, or those with a history of cerebellar symptoms post-CEA.

The surgical treatment of carotid artery stenosis demands a personalized and evidence-based approach. CEA remains the primary intervention for most patients, offering excellent long-term outcomes. However, CAS provides an alternative for high-risk individuals or those with anatomic anomalies. By carefully evaluating each patient's unique circumstances, adhering to established guidelines, and employing a multidisciplinary approach, surgeons can optimize outcomes, reduce complications, and enhance the quality of life for patients with carotid artery stenosis.

6. Non-surgical treatment

Non-surgical management of carotid artery stenosis is a comprehensive approach that integrates pharmacological therapy, lifestyle modifications, and risk factor management. The primary objectives of this approach are to stabilize atherosclerotic plaques, slow disease progression, and reduce the risk of cerebrovascular events. Treatment plans are tailored to the individual patient based on their unique clinical profile, comorbidities, and risk factors, with regular follow-up to assess treatment efficacy and response [52].

6.1 Medical therapy

Medical therapy serves as the cornerstone of non-surgical treatment for carotid artery stenosis, focusing on pharmacological interventions to mitigate risk factors, stabilize plaques, and prevent thrombotic complications.

6.1.1 Antiplatelet therapy

Antiplatelet agents are essential for reducing the risk of thrombus formation and subsequent cerebrovascular events [53].

- *Aspirin*: The first-line antiplatelet agent, with a daily dosage ranging from 75 to 100 mg. Aspirin is fundamental for stroke prevention, particularly in patients with carotid artery stenosis. It is often initiated at low doses to minimize gastrointestinal side effects.

- *Clopidogrel*: Administered daily at a dose of 75 mg, it is particularly useful for patients who are intolerant to aspirin or those at higher risk of thrombosis due to other cardiovascular risk factors. For patients with aspirin allergy or intolerance, alternative antiplatelet agents such as ticagrelor or prasugrel may be considered.

6.1.2 Statin therapy

Statins are pivotal for lipid management and plaque stabilization, playing a critical role in reducing cardiovascular risk [54].

- *LDL-C reduction*: The target is to achieve an LDL cholesterol level of 1.8 mmol/L (70 mg/dL) or a reduction of at least 50% from baseline. Commonly prescribed statins include atorvastatin, rosuvastatin, and simvastatin. These agents not only lower LDL cholesterol but also exhibit anti-inflammatory effects, contributing to plaque stabilization.

- *Plaque stabilization*: Statins inhibit the inflammatory processes within atherosclerotic plaques, reducing the likelihood of plaque rupture and subsequent thrombus formation. For patients who experience statin-induced myopathy, alternative medications such as pravastatin or red yeast rice may be explored.

6.1.3 Antihypertensive therapy

Hypertension is a major modifiable risk factor for cerebrovascular events. Management involves tailored antihypertensive therapy to achieve personalized blood pressure goals [55].

- *First-line agents*: Angiotensin-converting enzyme (ACE) inhibitors, angiotensin receptor blockers (ARBs), and calcium channel blockers (CCBs) are commonly utilized. The choice depends on the patient's comorbid conditions and tolerance.

- *Blood pressure targets*: The target systolic blood pressure (SBP) is generally <140 mmHg for most patients. For diabetic patients, a stricter target of <130 mmHg is advised. In elderly patients, a slightly higher target of <150 mmHg may be considered based on individual tolerance and comorbidities.

- *Polytherapy*: Combined antihypertensive regimens are often necessary to achieve target blood pressure. The selection of combination therapy is guided by the patient's response, side effect profiles, and potential drug interactions.

6.1.4 Antidiabetic therapy

Diabetes mellitus significantly increases the risk of atherosclerotic progression. Glycemic control is essential to reduce vascular complications and improve long-term outcomes [56].

- *Glycemic targets*: Fasting plasma glucose should be maintained below 7.0 mmol/L, with a hemoglobin A1c (HbA1c) goal of <7%. For patients with gestational diabetes or other specific conditions, individualized targets may be set.

- *Pharmacological management*: Metformin is the first-line medication for most diabetic patients, particularly those without contraindications. Additional agents such as sulphonylureas, DPP-4 inhibitors, GLP-1 receptor agonists, or insulin therapy are added based on individual glycemic response and comorbid conditions.

6.1.5 Other pharmacological agents

Additional medications may be employed based on specific patient conditions to address unique risk factors.

- *Anticoagulants*: Indications include patients with atrial fibrillation or other conditions requiring anticoagulation. Warfarin or novel oral anticoagulants (NOACs), such as dabigatran, rivaroxaban, or apixaban, may be prescribed. Close monitoring for bleeding risks is essential [57].

- *Antioxidants*: Agents such as vitamin C and vitamin E are sometimes used to mitigate oxidative stress, although their efficacy in reducing stroke risk remains inconclusive. Emerging evidence suggests limited benefits in this context [58].

- *Homocysteine management*: In patients with elevated homocysteine levels, supplementation with folic acid, vitamin B6, and B12 may be considered to reduce cardiovascular risk. This approach is particularly relevant in populations with genetic methylenetetrahydrofolate reductase (MTHFR) defects [59].

6.1.6 Smoking cessation support

Tobacco cessation is a critical component of cardiovascular risk reduction. Nicotine replacement therapy or pharmacological aids, such as varenicline or bupropion, may be prescribed to assist patients in quitting smoking. Behavioral therapy or support groups are often incorporated into smoking cessation programs to enhance success rates [60].

6.2 Lifestyle modifications

Lifestyle interventions are essential for managing carotid artery stenosis, complementing pharmacological therapy to reduce risk factors and improve vascular health.

6.2.1 Dietary modifications

A heart-healthy diet is fundamental for managing risk factors and promoting vascular health. The following dietary recommendations are emphasized [61]:

- *Mediterranean or DASH Diet*: Patients are advised to adopt a diet rich in fruits, vegetables, whole grains, fatty fish, and nuts. These dietary patterns are associated with reduced inflammation and improved vascular endothelial function.

- *Limit saturated and trans fats*: Patients are counseled to avoid trans fats and cholesterol-rich foods to reduce LDL cholesterol levels. This includes limiting processed foods, fried foods, and high-fat dairy products.

- *Sodium restriction*: A daily sodium intake of <2300 mg is recommended to help manage blood pressure. For individuals with hypertension, a further reduction to <1500 mg per day may be beneficial.

- *Personalized diet plans*: Cultural preferences and individual dietary restrictions are considered when creating personalized diet plans, ensuring adherence to heart-healthy principles.

6.2.2 Environment and carotid atherosclerosis

Emerging evidence highlights the role of environmental factors in the development and progression of carotid atherosclerosis, independent of traditional risk factors. Key environmental exposures include [62–65]:

- Air pollution: Particulate matter ($PM_{2.5}$ and PM_{10}) and traffic-related pollutants (e.g., nitrogen dioxide) are linked to endothelial dysfunction, systemic inflammation, and accelerated atherosclerosis. Long-term exposure is associated with increased carotid intima-media thickness (CIMT) and plaque formation.

- Nanoplastics and microplastics: These ubiquitous environmental contaminants may promote oxidative stress and vascular inflammation, though direct evidence in carotid atherosclerosis remains limited. Animal studies suggest nanoplastics exacerbate endothelial injury and lipid deposition.

- Heavy metals: Chronic exposure to lead, cadmium, and arsenic correlates with elevated cardiovascular risk, partly through oxidative damage and impaired nitric oxide bioavailability.

- Noise pollution: Chronic noise exposure (e.g., traffic and industrial) is tied to stress-mediated pathways, increasing cortisol and catecholamines, which may worsen vascular dysfunction.

6.2.3 Weight management

Excess adiposity is a significant risk factor for atherosclerosis. Weight loss is encouraged for patients who are overweight or obese, with a target body mass index (BMI) of 18.5–24.9 kg/m^2. Waist circumference goals include <90 cm for men and < 85 cm for women [66].

- *Dietary counseling*: Patients receive guidance on energy-restricted diets, portion control, and increasing physical activity to achieve weight loss goals.

- *Behavioral strategies*: Behavioral interventions, such as regular meal planning and tracking food intake, are recommended to enhance adherence to weight management plans.

6.2.4 Physical activity

Regular exercise is essential for improving cardiovascular health and reducing risk factors. The following recommendations are provided [67]:

- *Aerobic exercise*: Patients are encouraged to engage in at least 150 minutes of moderate-intensity aerobic activity per week, such as brisk walking, cycling, or swimming. For individuals with physical limitations, lower-intensity exercises or water-based activities are recommended.

- *Resistance training*: Incorporating strength training exercises 2–3 times per week helps enhance cardiovascular fitness and muscle strength. Resistance exercises may include bodyweight exercises, resistance bands, or machine-based workouts.

- *Exercise regimens*: Exercise programs are tailored to individual capabilities and preferences, ensuring compliance and long-term adherence.

6.2.5 Alcohol moderation

Excessive alcohol consumption increases the risk of hypertension and cardiovascular complications. Patients are advised to limit alcohol intake as follows [68]:

- *Men*: No more than 25 grams of alcohol per day (equivalent to 1–2 standard drinks).

- *Women*: No more than 15 grams of alcohol per day (equivalent to 1 standard drink).

6.2.6 Stress management and mental health

Chronic stress can exacerbate cardiovascular risk by increasing blood pressure and promoting atherosclerotic progression. Patients are encouraged to engage in stress-reduction activities, such as mindfulness, meditation, or yoga. Psychological support, including counseling or participation in support groups, may be beneficial for patients with anxiety or depression.

6.3 Regular follow-up and monitoring

Comprehensive follow-up and monitoring are essential to assess treatment response, detect disease progression, and optimize management plans.

6.3.1 Laboratory monitoring

- *Lipid profile*: Reassessed every 6–12 months to ensure LDL cholesterol goals are being met. This monitoring helps guide statin therapy adjustments and provides insights into overall cardiovascular risk.

- *Blood glucose*: Regular monitoring, particularly for diabetic patients, is crucial for optimizing glycemic control and preventing complications. HbA1c levels are measured quarterly or more frequently if needed.

- *Hematologic and renal function*: Patients on statins or antihypertensives require regular monitoring of liver function and renal function to identify potential side effects and ensure safe medication use.

6.3.2 Imaging surveillance

- *Cervical artery ultrasound*: Performed every 6–12 months to assess plaque morphology, thickness, and composition. This surveillance helps identify disease progression or stabilization and guides treatment adjustments.

- *Carotid artery duplex imaging*: Used to evaluate changes in blood flow velocities and detect new or worsening stenosis. This imaging modality is particularly useful for monitoring high-risk patients and those with recent cerebrovascular events.

6.3.3 Neurological assessments

- *Neurological evaluations*: Regularly conducted to detect signs of cerebrovascular events, such as transient ischemic attacks (TIAs) or silent strokes. This includes monitoring for new or worsening neurological symptoms, such as dizziness, visual disturbances, or cognitive changes.

- *Vascular risk stratification*: Periodic reassessment of cardiovascular risk factors, including lipid profiles, blood pressure, and glucose levels, helps guide ongoing management and prevent adverse events.

6.4 Patient education

Patient education is a cornerstone of effective management, empowering patients to actively participate in their care and adhere to treatment recommendations.

6.4.1 Disease awareness

Patients are educated about the nature of carotid artery disease, its potential complications, and the importance of adhering to prescribed therapies. Understanding the disease pathophysiology and the significance of risk factor modification enhances patient engagement.

6.4.2 Medication adherence

- *Medication regimens*: Patients receive clear instructions on the correct use of medications, including dosages, administration schedules, and potential side effects. This includes guidance on when and how to adjust medications under medical supervision.

- *Titration plans*: Patients are educated on how and when to initiate or adjust medications, particularly for drugs requiring titration, such as statins or antihypertensives. This ensures safe and effective therapy implementation.

6.4.3 Lifestyle modifications

- *Dietary recommendations*: Patients are provided with tailored dietary advice, including examples of heart-healthy meal plans and guidance on selecting nutrient-rich foods. Educational materials, such as handouts or meal prep guides, may be distributed.

- *Exercise routines*: Patients receive guidance on setting up an individualized exercise program, including examples of achievable activities and a suggested weekly schedule. Visual aids or written plans may enhance adherence.

- *Smoking cessation support*: Patients are provided with resources and strategies to quit smoking, such as nicotine replacement therapy, quit-smoking medications, and access to counseling services. Support groups or mobile health apps may be recommended for additional support.

6.4.4 Stroke warning signs

Education on identifying stroke symptoms is critical for timely intervention. Patients are instructed to seek immediate medical attention if they experience any of the following symptoms:

- Sudden confusion or difficulty understanding speech
- Sudden weakness or numbness on one side of the body
- Sudden difficulty with walking or coordination
- Sudden loss of vision or double vision
- Sudden severe headache with no known cause

Prompt recognition of these symptoms can significantly improve outcomes by enabling timely treatment.

6.4.5 Follow-up appointments

Patients are educated on the importance of keeping regular follow-up appointments for both clinical assessments and imaging studies. This ensures continuous monitoring of disease progression and treatment efficacy. Regular visits also provide an opportunity for treatment optimization and addressing any emerging concerns.

7. Discussion

7.1 Treatment of asymptomatic carotid artery stenosis

The management of asymptomatic carotid artery stenosis (ACS) remains a contentious issue in contemporary vascular medicine, with ongoing debates regarding the optimal treatment strategies. Historically, surgical interventions, particularly carotid endarterectomy (CEA), were regarded as superior to the best medical therapy (BMT) in mitigating the risk of cerebrovascular events. However, the emergence of carotid artery stenting (CAS) as a less invasive alternative has significantly expanded treatment options, prompting a comparative evaluation of CAS versus CEA.

Early epidemiological studies and clinical trials consistently demonstrated that CEA provided a substantial advantage over BMT in reducing stroke risk, with findings supported by multiple studies. The introduction of CAS, characterized by its minimally invasive nature and potential advantages in preserving endothelial function, has led to a comparative analysis of CAS versus CEA. Over the past decade, numerous randomized controlled trials (RCTs) have demonstrated that both CAS and CEA exhibit comparable efficacy and risk profiles, suggesting that treatment selection may be guided by patient-specific factors, surgeon expertise, and institutional practices [69].

Concomitant with advancements in surgical techniques, modern BMT regimens have undergone significant refinements, incorporating potent statins, antiplatelet agents, and comprehensive risk modification strategies. Notably, contemporary BMT has achieved a remarkably low annual stroke rate of approximately 0.9% in ACS patients managed conservatively [70]. This favorable outcome has led some investigators to speculate that, in certain patient populations, medical therapy alone may suffice, potentially obviating the need for surgical intervention. A recent meta-analysis comparing the efficacy of vascular reconstruction, traditional BMT (prior to 2000), and modern BMT (post-2000) revealed that, while CEA and CAS significantly reduced ischemic stroke rates compared to all BMT approaches, they did not exhibit superior outcomes compared to modern BMT [71]. This observation challenges the conventional paradigm and suggests that, under modern therapeutic regimens, medical therapy may rival surgical options in certain cases.

Despite these advancements, the debate persists, underscoring the need for further high-quality, large-scale RCTs. Such studies are essential to elucidate the relative benefits and risks of BMT, CAS, and CEA under contemporary treatment protocols thereby providing more robust evidence for clinical decision-making.

7.2 Intrastent restenosis in carotid artery stenosis

In the surgical management of carotid artery stenosis, both CEA and CAS present unique advantages and challenges. Notably, CAS has been associated with a higher incidence of intrastent restenosis (ISR) compared to CEA [72]. ISR, defined as a recurrent narrowing exceeding 50% within or adjacent to the stent, poses a critical risk of recurrent cerebrovascular events and undermines the long-term efficacy of the intervention. The pathophysiology of ISR is multifactorial, encompassing lipid abnormalities, diabetes mellitus, smoking history, stent design, and residual narrowing post-procedure. These factors collectively contribute to neointimal hyperplasia and vascular remodeling, which are central to ISR development.

Effective management of these modifiable risk factors is imperative to mitigate the likelihood of ISR. Treatment options for patients experiencing ISR include repeat CEA, CAS, stent retrieval, or carotid bypass surgery [73]. Pharmacological interventions, such as long-term antiplatelet therapy and statin use, play a critical role in reducing ISR risk by inhibiting platelet aggregation and reducing vascular inflammation [74].

Emerging therapeutic strategies are being explored to address ISR. Among these, the use of drug-eluting balloons (DEBs) has shown promise. DEBs, which incorporate medications such as paclitaxel or sirolimus to inhibit excessive cell proliferation, have demonstrated favorable results in reducing ISR rates. However, while initial studies suggest efficacy, the long-term clinical benefits of DEBs require further validation through extensive clinical follow-up [75]. Additionally, advancements in gene-editing technologies, such as CRISPR-Cas9, offer potential avenues for targeting lipid metabolism and slowing the progression of atherosclerosis. These technologies are currently in the experimental stage but hold promise for future therapeutic applications [76].

Looking forward, research should focus on elucidating the molecular mechanisms underlying ISR, with the ultimate goal of developing more effective preventive and therapeutic strategies. This includes investigations into the role of endothelial function, inflammatory mediators, and genetic predisposition in ISR development. Furthermore, the exploration of novel stent technologies, such as bioabsorbable stents and drug-eluting stents with advanced polymer platforms, may offer innovative solutions to the ISR challenge.

In conclusion, the treatment paradigm for asymptomatic carotid artery stenosis is continually evolving, driven by advancements in both surgical and medical therapies. While CEA and CAS remain viable options, the emergence of modern BMT challenges conventional treatment protocols. As the field progresses, a deeper understanding of ISR and the development of innovative therapies will be essential in optimizing treatment outcomes and enhancing the quality of life for patients with carotid artery stenosis. Continued collaboration among clinicians, researchers, and industry partners is imperative to address the remaining uncertainties and refine treatment strategies for ACS patients.

8. Conclusion

8.1 Carotid artery stenosis and its impact on public health

Carotid artery atherosclerotic stenosis represents a significant vascular condition, being one of the leading causes of ischemic stroke, a disease that imposes substantial public health challenges globally. This narrowing of the carotid artery, primarily due to atherosclerotic plaque buildup, poses a critical risk of stroke when plaques rupture, obstructing cerebral blood flow. The management of this condition is pivotal in reducing the incidence of ischemic stroke and improving patient outcomes.

8.2 Comprehensive diagnostic and risk assessment

Effective management of carotid artery stenosis begins with a thorough diagnostic evaluation. This involves a combination of clinical examination, imaging studies such as carotid ultrasound and angiography, and cardiovascular risk profiling. These assessments are crucial in determining the extent of stenosis and the patient's overall risk profile, guiding appropriate treatment decisions.

8.3 Treatment strategies: Individualized approaches

The treatment approach for carotid artery stenosis is inherently individualized, tailored to the patient's specific clinical presentation and comorbid conditions. For asymptomatic patients, particularly those at lower risk, medical therapy emerges as a cornerstone. This regimen typically includes statins to lower LDL cholesterol, antiplatelet agents to prevent thrombus formation, and comprehensive risk factor modification, such as lifestyle changes and blood pressure management.

In contrast, for high-risk symptomatic patients, surgical interventions such as carotid endarterectomy (CEA) or carotid artery stenting (CAS) may be more appropriate. The choice between these procedures depends on factors such as vascular anatomy, patient-specific risks, and the surgeon's expertise. Both CEA and CAS have their respective advantages and challenges, with CEA often preferred for its durability and CAS for its minimally invasive nature.

DOI: http://dx.doi.org/10.5772/intechopen.1010566

8.4 Emerging therapies and future directions

The field of vascular medicine is continually evolving, with emerging therapies offering promising avenues for improved patient outcomes. Among these, drug-eluting balloons (DEBs) and advanced stent technologies are gaining attention for their potential to reduce intrastent restenosis. These devices release medications like paclitaxel or sirolimus, inhibiting excessive cell proliferation within the stent. However, while preliminary studies demonstrate efficacy, further research is essential to establish their long-term benefits and safety across diverse patient populations.

Additionally, advancements in imaging modalities and a deeper understanding of the molecular mechanisms underlying atherosclerosis are paving the way for more precise and effective treatment strategies. These developments, coupled with ongoing research, hold the potential to refine therapeutic approaches and address current limitations.

8.5 Multidisciplinary approach and lifestyle modifications

The management of carotid artery stenosis demands a multidisciplinary approach that integrates medical, surgical, and lifestyle interventions. Lifestyle modifications, including dietary changes, regular physical activity, smoking cessation, and stress management, play a crucial role in risk reduction and disease management. Patient education is equally vital, empowering individuals to actively engage in their care and adhere to prescribed therapies.

In summary, the effective management of carotid artery stenosis requires a tailored, patient-centered approach that combines medical therapy, surgical options, and lifestyle interventions. By prioritizing comprehensive diagnostic evaluation and individualized treatment plans, clinicians can optimize patient outcomes, reduce the risk of stroke recurrence, and enhance quality of life. As the field advances, continued collaboration among researchers, clinicians, and healthcare providers is essential to address the complex challenges posed by carotid artery stenosis. Through ongoing innovation and research, the goal remains to further refine treatment strategies and ultimately reduce the global burden of ischemic stroke.

Acknowledgements

The authors acknowledge the use of DeepSeek for language polishing of the manuscript.

Fund

None.

Conflict of interest

Authors declare that they have no conflict of interest.

Notes/thanks/other declarations

None declared.

Ethics statement

This study was exempted from the review by the institutional ethics committee. This article does not include any information that may identify the person.

Author details

Changyang Zhong[1]*, Jingxin Zhang[1], Cong Wu[2], Yinquan Sun[3], Wei Zhu[3], Yong Lu[4], Huiming Dou[5], Guochu Peng[6] and Zhang Zuyong[7]

1 Cerebrovascular Disease Department, Hangzhou Third People's Hospital, Hangzhou, China

2 Zhejiang Chinese Medical University, Hangzhou, China

3 Hangzhou Hi-tech Industry Development Zone (Binjiang District) Bureau of Health, China

4 Hangzhou Binjiang District Puyan Street Community Health Service Center, China

5 Hangzhou Binjiang District Xixing Street Community Health Service Center, China

6 Hangzhou Binjiang District Changhe Street Community Health Service Center, China

7 Hangzhou Third People's Hospital, Hangzhou, China

*Address all correspondence to: zhonghening@163.com

References

[1] Katan M, Luft A. Global burden of stroke. Seminars in Neurology. 2018;**38**(2):208-211. DOI: 10.1055/s-0038-1649503. Epub 2018 May 23

[2] Lackland DT, Roccella EJ, Deutsch AF, et al. Factors influencing the decline in stroke mortality: A statement from the American Heart Association/American Stroke Association. Stroke. 2014;**45**(1):315-353

[3] Gupta A, Kesavabhotla K, Baradaran H, et al. Plaque echolucency and stroke risk in asymptomatic carotid stenosis: A systematic review and meta-analysis. Stroke. 2015;**46**(1):91-97

[4] Wang J, Qin S, Zhang X, et al. Identification of macrophage-associated novel drug targets in atherosclerosis based on integrated transcriptome features. Journal of Chemical Information and Modeling. 2024;**64**(23):9009-9020

[5] Mughal M, Khan MK, DeMarco JK, et al. Symptomatic and asymptomatic carotid artery plaque. Expert Review of Cardiovascular Therapy. 2011;**9**(10):1315-1330

[6] Wasserman BA. Clinical carotid atherosclerosis. Neuroimaging Clinics. 2002;**12**(3):403-419

[7] Sirven JI, Hastings JD, Wood SJ. Aerospace Neurology[J]. 5th ed. Fundamentals of Aerospace Medicine; 2021

[8] Banerjee C, Chimowitz MI. Stroke caused by atherosclerosis of the major intracranial arteries. Circulation Research. 2017;**120**(3):502-513

[9] Zarins CK, Giddens DP, Bharadvaj BK, et al. Carotid bifurcation atherosclerosis. Quantitative correlation of plaque localization with flow velocity profiles and wall shear stress. Circulation Research. 1983;**53**(4):502-514

[10] Zhang S, Liu Y, Cao Y, et al. Targeting the microenvironment of vulnerable atherosclerotic plaques: An emerging diagnosis and therapy strategy for atherosclerosis. Advanced Materials. 2022;**34**(29):2110660

[11] Libby P. Inflammation during the life cycle of the atherosclerotic plaque. Cardiovascular Research. 2021;**117**(13):2525-2536

[12] Miceli G, Basso MG, Pintus C, et al. Molecular pathways of vulnerable carotid plaques at risk of ischemic stroke: A narrative review. International Journal of Molecular Sciences. 2024;**25**(8):4351

[13] Caplan LR, Simon RP, Hassani S. Cerebrovascular disease—stroke[M]//Neurobiology of brain disorders. Academic Press; 2023:457-476

[14] Baaten C, Nagy M, Bergmeier W, et al. Platelet biology and function: Plaque erosion vs. rupture. European Heart Journal. 2024;**45**(1):18-31

[15] Seime T. The Role of Smooth Muscle Cells in Calcification of Atherosclerotic Plaques. Sweden: Karolinska Institutet; 2021

[16] Nichols W. Nature of Flow of a Liquid[M]//McDonald's Blood Flow in Arteries. CRC Press; 2022:25-67

[17] Trotman-Lucas M, Gibson CL. A review of experimental models of focal cerebral ischemia focusing on the middle cerebral artery occlusion model. F1000Research. 2021;**10**:242

[18] Kizhisseri M, Gharaie S, Boopathy SR, et al. Differential sensitivities to blood pressure variations in internal carotid and intracranial arteries: A numerical approach to stroke prediction. Scientific Reports. 2023;**13**(1):22319

[19] McGurgan IJ, Kelly PJ, Turan TN, et al. Long-term secondary prevention: Management of blood pressure after a transient ischemic attack or stroke. Stroke. 2022;**53**(4):1085-1103

[20] Li J, Somers VK, Gao X, et al. Evaluation of optimal diastolic blood pressure range among adults with treated systolic blood pressure less than 130 mm Hg. JAMA Network Open. 2021;**4**(2):e2037554

[21] Pacinella G, Ciaccio AM, Tuttolomondo A. Endothelial dysfunction and chronic inflammation: The cornerstones of vascular alterations in age-related diseases. International Journal of Molecular Sciences. 2022;**23**(24):15722

[22] Virdis A, Giannarelli C, Fritsch Neves M, et al. Cigarette smoking and hypertension. Current Pharmaceutical Design. 2010;**16**(23):2518-2525

[23] Poznyak AV, Sukhorukov VN, Surkova R, et al. Glycation of LDL: AGEs, impact on lipoprotein function, and involvement in atherosclerosis. Frontiers in Cardiovascular Medicine. 2023;**10**:1094188

[24] Adorni MP, Ronda N, Bernini F, et al. High density lipoprotein cholesterol efflux capacity and atherosclerosis in cardiovascular disease: Pathophysiological aspects and pharmacological perspectives. Cells. 2021;**10**(3):574

[25] Joglar JA, Chung MK, Armbruster AL, et al. 2023 ACC/AHA/ACCP/HRS guideline for the diagnosis and management of atrial fibrillation: A report of the American College of Cardiology/American Heart Association joint committee on clinical practice guidelines. Journal of the American College of Cardiology. 2024;**83**(1):109-279

[26] Jayawardena R, Sooriyaarachchi P, Misra A. Abdominal obesity and metabolic syndrome in South Asians: Prevention and management. Expert Review of Endocrinology & Metabolism. 2021;**16**(6):339-349

[27] Feingold KR. The effect of diet on cardiovascular disease and lipid and lipoprotein levels[J]. 2021

[28] Kong P, Cui ZY, Huang XF, et al. Inflammation and atherosclerosis: Signaling pathways and therapeutic intervention. Signal Transduction and Targeted Therapy. 2022;**7**(1):131

[29] Sherratt SCR, Libby P, Budoff MJ, et al. Role of omega-3 fatty acids in cardiovascular disease: The debate continues. Current Atherosclerosis Reports. 2023;**25**(1):1-17

[30] Sorout J, Kacker S, Saboo N. Metabolic syndrome and possible treatments (consecutive therapies): A literature review. International Journal of Endocrinology (Ukraine). 2022;**18**(6):351-357

[31] Vacca A, Bulfone L, Cicco S, et al. Alcohol intake and arterial hypertension: Retelling of a multifaceted story. Nutrients. 2023;**15**(4):958

[32] Strauss MH, Hall AS, Narkiewicz K. The combination of beta-blockers and ACE inhibitors across the spectrum of cardiovascular diseases. Cardiovascular Drugs and Therapy. 2023;**37**(4):757-770

[33] Marx N, Husain M, Lehrke M, et al. GLP-1 receptor agonists for the reduction of atherosclerotic cardiovascular risk in patients with type 2 diabetes. Circulation. 2022;**146**(24):1882-1894

[34] Bonati LH, Kakkos S, Berkefeld J, et al. European stroke organisation guideline on endarterectomy and stenting for carotid artery stenosis. European Stroke Journal. 2021;**6**(2):I-XLVII

[35] Saba L, Scicolone R, Johansson E, et al. Quantifying carotid stenosis: History, current applications, limitations, and potential: How imaging is changing the scenario. Life. 2024;**14**(1):73

[36] Miceli G, Basso MG, Pintus C, et al. Molecular pathways of vulnerable carotid plaques at risk of ischemic stroke: A narrative review. International Journal of Molecular Sciences. 2024;**25**(8):4351

[37] Busto G, Morotti A, Carlesi E, et al. Pivotal role of multiphase computed tomography angiography for collateral assessment in patients with acute ischemic stroke. La Radiologia Medica. 2023;**128**(8):944-959

[38] Gać P, Jakubowska-Martyniuk A, Żórawik A, et al. Diagnostic methods of atherosclerotic plaque and the assessment of its prognostic significance—A narrative review. Journal of Cardiovascular Development and Disease. 2024;**11**(11):343

[39] Mendelson SJ, Prabhakaran S. Diagnosis and management of transient ischemic attack and acute ischemic stroke: A review. JAMA. 2021;**325**(11):1088-1098

[40] Mergenthaler P, Dirnagl U, Kunz A. Ischemic stroke: Basic pathophysiology and clinical implication. In: Neuroscience in the 21st Century: From Basic to Clinical. Cham: Springer International Publishing; 2022. pp. 3807-3827

[41] Tuna MA, Rothwell PM. Diagnosis of non-consensus transient ischaemic attacks with focal, negative, and non-progressive symptoms: Population-based validation by investigation and prognosis. The Lancet. 2021;**397**(10277):902-912

[42] Parkkila K, Kiviniemi A, Tulppo M, et al. Carotid and femoral bruits as cardiovascular risk indicators in a middle-aged Finnish population: A 20-year prospective study. PLoS One. 2022;**17**(12):e0278901

[43] Wang T, Xu X, et al. Association between fundus atherosclerosis and carotid arterial atherosclerosis. International Journal of Clinical Medicine. 2023;**14**(5):282-289

[44] Cassola N, Baptista-Silva JC, Nakano LCU, et al. Duplex ultrasound for diagnosing symptomatic carotid stenosis in the extracranial segments[J]. Cochrane Database of Systematic Reviews. 2022;(7)

[45] Saba L, Antignani PL, Gupta A, et al. International Union of Angiology (IUA) consensus paper on imaging strategies in atherosclerotic carotid artery imaging: From basic strategies to advanced approaches. Atherosclerosis. 2022;**354**:23-40

[46] Saxena A, Ng EYK, Lim ST. Imaging modalities to diagnose carotid artery stenosis: Progress and prospect. Biomedical Engineering Online. 2019;**18**:1-23

[47] van der Vaart MG, Meerwaldt R, Reijnen MMPJ, et al. Endarterectomy or carotid artery stenting: The quest continues. The American Journal of Surgery. 2008;**195**(2):259-269

[48] Naylor R, Rantner B, Ancetti S, et al. Editor's choice—European Society for Vascular Surgery (ESVS) 2023 clinical practice guidelines on the management of atherosclerotic carotid and vertebral artery disease. European Journal of Vascular and Endovascular Surgery. 2023;**65**(1):7-111

[49] White CJ, Brott TG, Gray WA, et al. Carotid artery stenting: JACC state-of-the-art review. Journal of the American College of Cardiology. 2022;**80**(2):155-170

[50] Heck D, Jost A. Carotid stenosis, stroke, and carotid artery revascularization. Progress in Cardiovascular Diseases. 2021;**65**:49-54

[51] Loftus CM, Kuroda S, Kuwayama N. Carotid Treatment: Principles and Techniques. CRC Press; 2023

[52] Piechocki M, Przewłocki T, Pieniążek P, et al. A non-coronary, peripheral arterial atherosclerotic disease (carotid, renal, lower limb) in elderly patients—A review: Part I—Epidemiology, risk factors, and atherosclerosis-related diversities in elderly patients. Journal of Clinical Medicine. 2024;**13**(5):1471

[53] Greco A, Occhipinti G, Giacoppo D, et al. Antithrombotic therapy for primary and secondary prevention of ischemic stroke: JACC state-of-the-art review. Journal of the American College of Cardiology. 2023;**82**(15):1538-1557

[54] Kadoglou NPE, Khattab E, Velidakis N, et al. A new approach of statin therapy in carotid atherosclerosis: Targeting indices of plaque vulnerability on the top of lipid-lowering. A narrative review. Polish Heart Journal (Kardiologia Polska). 2022;**80**(9):880-890

[55] Kivipelto M, Palmer K, Hoang TD, et al. Trials and treatments for vascular brain health: Risk factor modification and cognitive outcomes. Stroke. 2022

[56] Antoniou S, Naka KK, Papadakis M, et al. Effect of glycemic control on markers of subclinical atherosclerosis in patients with type 2 diabetes mellitus: A review. World Journal of Diabetes. 2021;**12**(11):1856

[57] Abdullah HM, Ullah W, Jafar MS, et al. Safety and efficacy of apixaban, rivaroxaban, and warfarin in end-stage renal disease with atrial fibrillation: A systematic review and meta-analysis. Cardiovascular Revascularization Medicine. 2021;**30**:26-32

[58] Schneider A. The Controversy around Vitamin E Supplementation: A Potential Treatment for Type 2 Diabetes-Related Oxidative Stress?. 2021

[59] Gospodarczyk A, Marczewski K, Gospodarczyk N, et al. Homocysteine and cardiovascular disease—A current review. Wiadomości Lekarskie. 2022;**75**(11 pt 2):2862-2866

[60] Baker TB, Piper ME, Smith SS, et al. Effects of combined varenicline with nicotine patch and of extended treatment duration on smoking cessation: A randomized clinical trial. JAMA. 2021;**326**(15):1485-1493

[61] Diab A, Dastmalchi LN, Gulati M, et al. A heart-healthy diet for cardiovascular disease prevention: Where are we now? Vascular Health and Risk Management. 2023:237-253

[62] Franklin BA, Brook R, Pope CA 3rd. Air pollution and cardiovascular disease. Current Problems in Cardiology. 2015;**40**(5):207-238

[63] Vethaak AD, Legler J. Microplastics and human health. Science. 2021;**371**(6530):672-674

[64] Münzel T, Steven S, Frenis K, et al. Environmental factors such as noise and air pollution and vascular disease. Antioxidants & Redox Signaling. 2020;**33**(9):581-601

[65] Rajagopalan S, Al-Kindi SG, Brook RD. Air pollution and cardiovascular disease. Journal of the American College of Cardiology. 2018;**72**(17):2054-2070

[66] Lopez-Jimenez F, Almahmeed W, Bays H, et al. Obesity and cardiovascular disease: Mechanistic insights and management strategies. A joint position paper by the world heart federation and world obesity federation. European Journal of Preventive Cardiology. 2022;**29**(17):2218-2237

[67] Kaminsky LA, German C, Imboden M, et al. The importance of healthy lifestyle behaviors in the prevention of cardiovascular disease. Progress in Cardiovascular Diseases. 2022;**70**:8-15

[68] Briasoulis A, Agarwal V, Messerli FH. Alcohol consumption and the risk of hypertension in men and women: A systematic review and meta-analysis. The Journal of Clinical Hypertension. 2012;**14**(11):792-798

[69] Musialek P, Bonati LH, Bulbulia R, et al. Stroke risk management in carotid atherosclerotic disease: A clinical consensus statement of the ESC Council on stroke and the ESC working group on aorta and peripheral vascular diseases. Cardiovascular Research. 2023:cvad135

[70] Loftus CM, Kuroda S, Kuwayama N. Carotid Treatment: Principles and Techniques. CRC Press; 2023

[71] Gasior SA, O'Donnell JPM, Davey M, et al. Optimal management of asymptomatic carotid artery stenosis: A systematic review and network meta-analysis. European Journal of Vascular and Endovascular Surgery. 2023;**65**(5):690-699

[72] Annamária M. Endovascular Treatment of Carotid In-Stent Restenosis. 2024

[73] Hrbáč T, Fiedler J, Procházka V, et al. Comparison of carotid endarterectomy and repeated carotid angioplasty and stenting for in-stent restenosis (CERCAS trial): A randomised study. Stroke and Vascular Neurology. 2023;**8**(5)

[74] Yang M, Kholmukhamedov A. Platelet reactivity in dyslipidemia: Atherothrombotic signaling and therapeutic implications. Reviews in Cardiovascular Medicine. 2021;**22**(1):67-81

[75] Wańha W, Bil J, Januszek R, et al. Long-term outcomes following drug-eluting balloons versus thin-strut drug-eluting stents for treatment of in-stent restenosis (DEB-dragon-registry). Circulation: Cardiovascular Interventions. 2021;**14**(9):e010868

[76] Alradwan I, Al Fayez N, Alomary MN, et al. Emerging trends and innovations in the treatment and diagnosis of atherosclerosis and cardiovascular disease: A comprehensive review towards healthier aging. Pharmaceutics. 2024;**16**(8):1037